COVID-19: LOCKDOWNS ON TRIAL

Michael Betrus

TABLE OF CONTENTS

INTRODUCTION

When COVID-19 first broke news in China, few saw it impacting America as a healthcare crisis. Initially the worst-case outlook was economic in nature – what will happen to our economy as American businesses are so entangled with China?

As the Grand Princess docked in Oakland in March, it seemed scary. What will the outcome be? Then something happened. Nothing. There was not a sweeping toll of hospitalizations and deaths. As we rolled into March and businesses shut down, followed by state lockdowns and unfathomable unemployment, I took serious notice. I began studying the cruise ship data trying to reconcile how that fit with crazy model projections that prompted the lockdowns.

Inside we recap in detail how COVID-19 began in China and spread across the world. We take a deep dive into the two quarantined cruise ships that provided invaluable data on the spread of the virus, who was affected and vulnerable, and what happened. On the cruise ships, we see that many passengers caught the virus and few were affected and far fewer still suffered a fatality as a result. We then deep dive into the models that prompted the lockdowns and reconcile them with the early cruise ship data.

Following that analysis, as the lockdowns began and gained momentum, we review what happened in many countries, including those in the European Union, Japan, South Korea and India. We look at each state, their impacts, hospitalizations and deaths. New York was particularly impacted in a way no other area in America was, and we dissect what happened there, as well as nursing homes around the country.

As we look at the growing number of COVID-19 deaths in America, many were counted *with* COVID-19 or *maybe* with COVID-19 but not necessarily dying *from* COVID-19, thus lowering the integrity of the data. Therefore, what was the impact on overall all-cause mortality? We look at total deaths in 2020 against the previous average, and we see a much lower number than what is reported. This is the single most important data point in measuring the impact of COVID-19.

The media has played the pivotal role in how the lockdowns have been engineered, as well as other policies like mandatory face masks. Are these appropriate measures? We take an in-depth look at how many in the media have inaccurately represented what has happened throughout the impact. Finally, what has happened as a result of the lockdowns? Schools closed, 40MM Americans out of work, deaths of despair like suicides and overdoses rising. Many consequential things happened as a result of the lockdowns and disproportionate to the actual risk.

I've written over a dozen career reference books and often conduct workshops for people to help them with their resumes, interviewing, anything to help them further their career. I get LinkedIn messages from around the world requesting help and it's always my highest priority, and I do all that consulting for free. A satisfying career is right up there with health and family in providing one fulfillment. Seeing the high unemployment triggered this research and the conclusions I've drawn.

This book is dedicated to those that lost their lives to COVID-19, particularly those helpless that passively contracted COVID-19 in care facilities where they and their families had to feel it was a protected environment. That included one of my family members in Detroit. It is also dedicated to the tens of millions of Americans and billions worldwide that have faced economic hardship over the COVID-19 lockdowns. Here the lockdowns are on trial. You be the judge.

CHAPTER 1

RECENT PANDEMIC HISTORY

Pandemic – *occurring over a wide geographic area and affecting an exceptionally high proportion of the population[1]*

According to the Centers for Disease Control (CDC), a pandemic "is a global outbreak of disease. Pandemics happen when a new virus emerges to infect people and can spread between people sustainably. Because there is little to no pre-existing immunity against the new virus, it spreads worldwide."

Within the life of anyone alive today, spanning back up to three generations, HIV/AIDS has by far been our biggest pandemic. It spans nearly all countries, has infected 75MM people, and 32MM people have died while possessing HIV.[2] This number will vary depending on the source. Anyone dying while possessing HIV is classified as dying of HIV for these statistics.

This distinction of how we classify deaths is critical for later consideration. Important to HIVs classification as a pandemic, infection resulting in serious illness to death, is that it is not an infliction that makes one segment of the population more vulnerable than another. HIV does not discriminate, whether you are healthy, young, old, a man or woman. For a patient with previous health underlying conditions, HIV has certainly proven to be more lethal. Without modern treatments it would also be lethal for otherwise healthy people.

Over the page there is a list of pandemics documented since the 20th century, some with staggering impacts on lives and societies.

THE SPANISH FLU

Where the Spanish Flu originated is questionable. Some suggest it emerged from soldiers returning from France in WWI and arriving in Kansas in early 1918. Hundreds of soldiers at Fort Riley, KS fell ill from flu-like symptoms.[3] It seemed to pass and some of those soldiers went on the Europe, where the virus mutated and became deadly. From those soldiers, the disease spread in Europe and ravaged populations across the world. WWI soldiers returned to America and in the fall of 1918, it spread like a wildfire. Some speculate the disease originated in China and was brought to North America from Chinese laborers in cramped trains traveling across Canada or supporting Chinese in WWI front lines in France.[4]

The Spanish Flu, the H1N1 virus, swept across the world from 1918-1919, claiming up to 50MM lives.[5] No vaccine existed, nor antibiotics, unlike today, which made treating secondary bacterial infections an ultimate game changer. It was most deadly for a sixteen-week period in the last quarter of 1918. According to the CDC, up to 500MM people were infected, about a third of the world's population at the time. In the United States, it claimed approximately 675,000 lives. Unique vulnerable age clusters varied from typical flu victim demographics. It's worth calling out that twice the number of Americans died from the Spanish Flu than from the battlefields of WWI.

The Spanish Flu claimed a high proportion of infected very young children, and then spiked up dramatically for those age 20-40 (see below). Unique to flu viruses is that the older you got, the less vulnerable to H1N1 you were, until you were over 80 and then the mortality rates skyrocketed.[6] It does not appear any source is certain why, other than as one aged they developed a kind of antibody immunity based on previous mild inflictions of variant strains of this virus. Most deaths attributed to the Spanish Flu were in people under age 65. Author John Barry cited in *The Great Influenza* that the single most vulnerable group of victims were pregnant women.

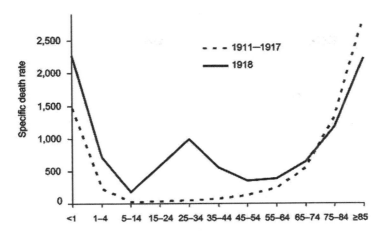

Source: Taubenberger, Jeffery K.; Morens, David M. (2006). "1918 Influenza: the Mother of All Pandemics".
Emerging Infectious Diseases. 12 (1): 15–22. doi:10.3201/eid1201.050979. PMC 3291398. PMID 16494711

When the Spanish Flu reached Boston, it began with soldiers in nearby Camp Devins. One soldier was misdiagnosed with it, and then spread it to a dozen soldiers within a day or two. Soon after a soldier contracted it, "he began to turn blue from a loss of oxygen and it is only a matter of a few hours then until death comes."[7] It took decades for the cause of the virus to be isolated and a vaccine developed to combat future outbreaks.

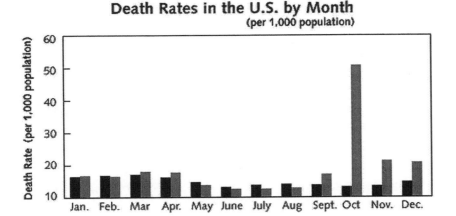

Source: https://employees.csbsju.edu/hjakubowski/classes/Chem%20and%20Society/Influenza/1918%20Pandemic.htm

It's shocking looking back at how the Spanish Flu ravaged through the country. Not long after, herd immunity was developed for survivors and it disappeared. For context on the chart above, consider that COVID-19 is lethal to about 2-3 per thousand infected people. The Spanish Flu reached 50 at its peak.

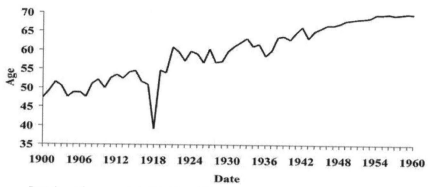

Figure above: Life expectancy in the United States, 1900–60, showing the impact of the 1918 influenza pandemic (Grove and Hetzel 1968; Linder and Grove 1943; United States Department of Commerce 1976).

Above is a chart of life expectancy in America, and the average age dip in 1918 is incomprehensible today to imagine. Below is a chart of several countries, their populations in 1918 and deaths attributed to the Spanish Flu. In reviewing dozens of sources and articles, death counts vary wildly, and the death numbers below are averages of what appeared to be the most reliable sources.

1918-1919 SPANISH FLU IMPACTS

COUNTRY	POPULATION	DEATHS
India	250,000,000	15,000,000
United States	103,000,000	675,000
Germany	65,000,000	426,000
Japan	58,000,000	360,000
England	42,000,000	220,000
France	39,000,000	400,000
Italy	36,000,000	410,000
Sweden	5,800,000	35,0000

UNITED STATES ACTIONS

There is an interesting and tragic story about when the Spanish Flu broke out in Philadelphia.[8] Public Health Director Wilmer Krusen was allegedly aware of an outbreak of a serious flu with soldiers returning from the war to Philadelphia. A large parade was planned for September 28, 1918, and Krusen declined to have it cancelled. Within three days of the parade, each of Philadelphia's hospitals were full and days later 2,800 people had died. The Spanish Flu was a wildfire in Philadelphia. On a single day more than 700 people died from that outbreak.

In contrast, according to Dave Roos of the History Channel, St. Louis and San Francisco made more aggressive efforts to stave off the contagion. Schools were shut down, public gatherings were stunted, many people wore gauze masks (later proved to not be of much help), and these two cities had a much lower death rate than Philadelphia. San Francisco was hit later, in early 1919, with a third wave and it proved very lethal.

According to Roos, many people protested against the masks and ban of public gatherings when not much happened, and the third time around they were hit very hard. It reads as if San Francisco and St. Louis early on practiced what nearly all cities and states were doing in the spring of 2020 to stave off COVID-19.

By 1919 the Spanish Flu was winding down and had nearly disappeared. The death rates vary from source to source, but by any measure it was the most merciless pandemic anyone alive at that time had seen. Some distinguishing qualifiers of the Spanish Flu pandemic:

- Highly contagious, likely airborne and certainly transmitted by contact
- Prompted pneumonia, often as a cause of death
- Impacted the world in a fairly short time (months) largely facilitated by WWI
- Caused death in otherwise healthy people, did not rely on underlying conditions
- Impacted multiple age brackets (very young, 20-40, over 80)

One thing that is so different between the Spanish Flu and COVID-19 is that COVID-19 preyed almost exclusively on the elderly and those with pre-existing conditions. The Spanish Flu killed the very young, men and women at their strongest (20-40), and then the very elderly.

HIV/AIDS

Since the Spanish Flu, the largest impacting pandemic has been the spread of the human immunodeficiency virus, or HIV. Unlike the Spanish Flu virus and COVID-19, HIV is spread through the exchange of bodily fluids: blood, semen, vaginal fluids. HIV has claimed over 26MM lives since its discovery in the late 1970s.

It was likely in existence since the mid-20th century in Africa. It may have been sourced from using chimpanzee tissue to grow polio vaccines where some of those chimpanzees carried Simian Immunodeficiency Virus (SIV). When the vaccines were extracted, they brought a new pathogen with them. Another theory is that it was sourced from the consumption of chimpanzee meat or from a mixing of chimpanzee blood with human blood in a victim one scenario.

HIV probably received little early attention and research funding because it was characterized as a disease transferred between gay male sexuality (mostly true early on in western countries) and drug users sharing intravenous needles. In 1990, an 18-year-old boy named Ryan White died from AIDS sourced from a blood transfusion. It sparked another level of fear and danger because before that, it wasn't factored that blood used for transfusions would be a source. But it was for him and Arthur Ashe, tennis great and humanitarian.

When Earvin "Magic" Johnson announced in 1991 he was HIV-positive, it brought HIV awareness and consideration well into the mainstream. Since then, treatments have improved to the point where, with treatment, most can realize such a low level of HIV in the blood that it is not measurable and not likely transferable.

HIV is a different type of virus than ones like H1N1 or COVID-19 but bears similar pandemic-characteristics to the Spanish Flu:

- Caused death in otherwise healthy people, did not rely on underlying conditions
- Impacted multiple age brackets
- No noted favoring of gender or race

UNITED STATES ACTIONS

HIV has had very high awareness in the United States for more than thirty years. People began practicing safer sex and drug users were less apt to share intravenous needles. No official social or economic policies changed to control HIV.

Treatments evolved since the 1990's have muted the virus before it affects the immune system to where today the survival rate is very high.

ASIAN FLU

The Asian Flu was first documented in Singapore and later Hong Kong in early 1957, where it then spread throughout China. It reached the west coast of the United States that summer, unnoticed at first. By November 1957, it had a huge impact, spreading and compromising health mostly in pregnant women, children and the elderly. Unlike the Spanish Flu, young men were not a major impacted segment.

By March 1958, nearly 70,000 Americans had died from the Asian Flu. Worldwide estimates vary from one to three million lives lost.

Interestingly, Dr. Maurice Hilleman was a microbiologist and former developer at what is now Bristol-Myers Squibb and a former leader of the Department of Respiratory Diseases at Army Medical Center (now the Walter Reed Army Institute of Research). He read about the Asian Flu breakout in 1957 and recognized it as a pandemic. He saw there was little immunity to the virus in America and drove the research and development of a vaccine.

Hilleman died in 2005 and is credited with developing many vaccines, including one for Hepatitis B, a precedent version of the one used today. Had Hilleman not caught it early on and drove the vaccine development for the Asian Flu, it may have impacted America like the Spanish Flu.

Pandemic characteristics of the Asian Flu include:

- Highly contagious, likely airborne and certainly transmitted by contact
- World-wide spread within several months
- Caused death in otherwise healthy people, did not rely on underlying conditions
- Impacted multiple age brackets (very young, pregnant women, the elderly)
- No noted favoring of gender or race

UNITED STATES ACTIONS

No social or economic policies changed over controlling the spread of the Asian Flu.

HONG KONG FLU

The Hong Kong Flu was the third influenza pandemic of the 20th century, believed to be a variant strain from the Asian Flu from a decade earlier. It is thought that people who survived the Asian Flu through antibodies present or the vaccine were immune to this one, a reason it was much less impacting than the Spanish Flu. The virus first took hold in Hong Kong in 1968, spread all over Southeast Asia quickly, and was brought to America by soldiers returning home from Vietnam.

The most vulnerable victims of the Hong Kong Flu were the very young and the elderly. That the Asian Flu and Hong Kong Flu originated in China is an interesting observation given where SARS-CoV-2 originated.

An estimated 100,000 people died of the Hong Kong Flu in America. At that time, the population in America was about 200 million people. That equates to .05% fatalities of all Americans. If the COVID-19 pandemic reaches that level, it would kill 160,000 Americans. I asked many people over seventy years old about the Hong Kong Flu and the only one who even remembered it was my uncle, a retired history teacher.

Pandemic characteristics of the Hong Kong Flu include:

- Highly contagious, likely airborne and certainly transmitted by contact
- World-wide spread within several months
- Caused death in the more vulnerable age groups of very young and elderly

UNITED STATES ACTIONS

No social or economic policies changed to control the spread of the Hong Kong Flu. No schools closed, no flights were cancelled, and nothing socially or economically changed. In fact, during the pandemic, a group of youths got together practicing whatever the opposite of social distancing was at a concert known as Woodstock on a farm in upstate New York. No federal intervention nor bailouts occurred. Life went on and if you ask Americans over 65 about it, most needed their memories jogged to even remember it, if they did at all.

SARS

Severe Acute Respiratory Syndrome (SARS), is based on a coronavirus first discovered in southern China in 2002 and thought to be sourced from bats. No significant number of deaths arose from SARS (800 worldwide), and the symptoms and illness cycle resemble the COVID-19 illness cycle.

UNITED STATES ACTIONS

No social or economic policies changed over controlling the spread of SARS.

SWINE FLU

The swine flu is a H1N1 virus-based influenza, similar to that of the Spanish Flu and is currently preventable with a vaccine. It did spread worldwide in 2009-2010 and is estimated that perhaps one billion people contracted it. With fewer than 250,000 worldwide deaths attributed to it, it had a milder impact than most flu seasons worldwide and in America.

UNITED STATES ACTIONS

No social or economic policies changed over controlling the spread of the Swine Flu.

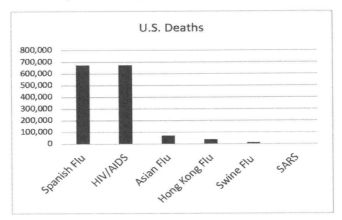

In a hundred years, the United States has been fortunate, more fortunate than many other countries, to have realized only two major pandemics: the Spanish Flu and HIV/AIDS. Noteworthy is that the HIV/AIDS pandemic has been slow moving and largely controllable, not easily spread and now very treatable. Many have feared that the COVID-19 threat to America and the world would mirror the Spanish Flu.

CHAPTER 2

INFLUENZA

Pandemics mentioned appropriately garner much note in history. Less attention is drawn to influenza infections each year. In recent years, flu shots have been available to lessen the blow, though the number of annual deaths surprises anyone unfamiliar with the data.

Flu viruses are different than SARS viruses. Both are infectious prompts to respiratory illness and pneumonia. Both cause similar symptoms: fever, body aches, cough, and may evolve into pneumonia. Flus may be caused by many different viruses. COVID-19 is caused by one, new and with no vaccine available at the time of the outbreak. Transmission is about the same. A bad flu season might kill 750,000 worldwide in a year, and as of June 2020 COVID-19 has taken more than 300,000 lives.

COVID-19 has demonstrated worse effects on Americans than our typical flu, much worse to a smaller segment of typical flu victims. The value in visiting flu case/death data is to put the COVID-19 impacts in some sort of context or perspective we're accustomed to. That scale is important when balanced with the extreme efforts many countries took to temper the hospitalization and death impacts, shutting down the world in ways never before seen in history.

The CDC estimates that since 2010, each year, anywhere from nine to forty-five million Americans are infected and get ill from the flu, a huge range and absolute number. Of that, between 140,000 and 800,000 people are hospitalized per year, and of that anywhere from 12,000 to more than 80,000 die. It's an astounding number that goes largely unnoticed by Americans, the media and politicians.

It also provides some degree of a benchmark of what is "acceptable" as a part of life and illness and death. That is not to say any death is "acceptable." My mom and her husband are 88 and live in Detroit. Each flu season, and particularly the coronavirus-impacted 2020, we drove home extra precautions. What is "acceptable" leads to when do we aggressively change behaviors, like lockdown society and the economy, to try to circumvent a viral disease?

December, January and March are about equal months in average influenza infections, hospitalizations and deaths, while on average February more than doubles any of those single months. The worst flu season in America in that span was the winter of 2017-2018. I caught it twice in 2018, traveling almost weekly, in both January and June of all times, and that after getting a flu shot in November of 2017.

Around 80,000 people died that flu season, a staggering amount. Were you aware of that? Neither was I. As a daily follower of several mainstream and smaller media outlets in print/online and cable news, I don't recall it mentioned. It surely was but since it did not make pronounced headlines, who really pays attention? More than 800,000 people were hospitalized, and the actual people infected, people like me who were not hospitalized, had to be in the tens of millions.

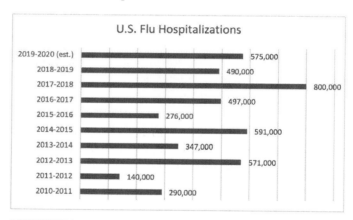

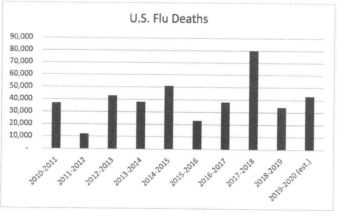

The noteworthy statistic here is the large number of hospitalizations and deaths associated with the flu each year. Even the bad 2017-2018 flu season did not warrant any policy or social change. Below is a list of influenza-related deaths by select states according to the CDC, in 2017 and an additional 50% increase to estimate the 2017-2018 flu season.[9]

The 2017-2018 flu season claimed twice the deaths as the previous year, with the peak in the first quarter of 2018. Conservatively, adding 2017 actuals with an additional fifty percent is a reasonable estimate where state-by-state data for that flu season is not readily available. The reason for adding fifty percent is that the 2017-2018 flu season killed twice the number from the previous year.

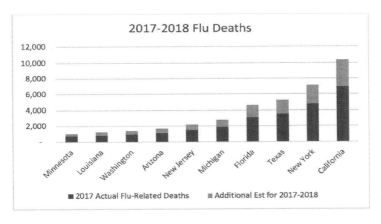

The chart above provides some context as we visit COVID-19 impacts per state later.

FLUS AROUND THE WORLD

ITALY

The International Journal of Infectious Diseases published a detailed analysis of influenza-impacted deaths in Italy in August 2019, compiled by several authors. In it, the report calls out that Italy has a higher than average elderly population. As a baseline, the population in Italy in 2017 was 60,000,000, about the same as California and Florida combined. Around 23% of Italy's population is over 65; California is closer to 12% and Florida, not surprisingly higher, is about 20%. On average, between 2013-2017, Italy lost 17,000 people annually to flu-related illnesses. COVID-19 would better than double that in 2020.

SWEDEN
Sweden's population is just over 10,000,000 people (the size of Michigan) with about 20% over 65 years old. In the 2017-2018 flu season, about 21,000 were confirmed with a flu diagnosis and of that, about a thousand died within a month of their diagnosis. Nearly all were over 65 years old.

SPAIN
Spain's population in 2018 was just over 46,000,000 (little bit bigger than California) and just over 18% of that are people over the age of 65. Spain lists about 12,000 flu-deaths in 2017-2018, considered one of their worst ever. Spain would lose more than 30,000 people to COVID-19 in 2020.

FRANCE
France's population in 2018 was just over 58,000,000, with 20% over 65 years old. In the 2014-2015 flu season, 18,000 lives were lost, a higher than average number for France. That is incredibly high, much higher as a percent of the population than the United States in our awful 2017-2018 flu season. COVID-19 would claim more than 30,000 lives in France in 2020.

ENGLAND
England's population in 2018 was 56,000,000 and of that, 18% were over 65 years old. For the 2017-2018 winter flu season, about 15,000 lives were lost, twice the average. That is a very high number, proportionately higher than the 80,000 flu deaths in America in the same flu season. The UK would lose more than 35,000 people to COVID-19 in 2020.

GERMANY
Germany had a population of nearly 83,000,000 people in 2018 with 20% over 65. According to the *General-Anzeiger*, in January 2018, in the 2014-2015 flu season, more than 21,000 deaths were due to flu-related illnesses. That ratio is about identical to the high infection year in America in 2017-2018. In a 2005 report, the U.S. National Library of Medicine-National Institutes of Health lists German flu deaths at conservatively 10 per 100,000 people, a rate much higher than the United States' highest death rates.

INDIA
India is the second most populated country at 1.4B. Of that, a very low 6% is over 65

years old. When we look at low flu death rates and COVID-19-related deaths, this will help to explain the very low percentages. In 2015 when the Swine Flu broke out, 2,000 people died from it. Generally, India reports low numbers for flu-related deaths, whether due to climate, younger age population or perhaps bad data.

AUSTRALIA
Australia has a population of about 25,000,000 and of that, nearly 16% are over 65. According to the Australian Bureau of Statistics, 1,255 people died from flu-related causes in 2017. The number triples if you include pneumonia, but under the influenza classification it is much lower. That ratio places it in the range of a mild flu impact in America any given year. One difference in their counting appears to be that they classify a death from influenza if that is the only cause, where in America often it is counted if they had it but perhaps also had another condition.

BRAZIL
The population in Brazil is 210,000,000 and 9% of that is over 65 years old. According to the U.S. National Library of Medicine-National Institutes of Health, Brazil realizes about one flu death per 100,000 people per year, or on average 2,100 deaths per year. This is very low compared to other countries. One suggested reasoning is the where Brazil resides in latitude. Perhaps that is a contributor to lower flu-related deaths in Australia and India, both inside their Tropic latitudes compared to other countries discussed here.

SOUTH KOREA
South Korea's population is about 52,000,000 and 14.5% of those people are over 65 years old. The Journal of Preventive Medicine and Public Health reports that on average, South Korea has 5,313 flu-associated deaths, with over 85% of those over 65 years old. That rate places South Korea below the United States.

Influenza-associated deaths in individual states, the United States as a whole and select other countries, provide the closest scale we can use as a benchmark of what "normal" or "acceptable" is in viral-prompted deaths. That's not to say that even one is acceptable; society, our norms, our government and history have dictated what is normal and acceptable. We all have accepted that 38,000 people die in car accidents per year. We know this is accepted because it's never talked about (I had to look it up) and no life-changing policies are in place (ever-improving safety standards notwithstanding).

CHAPTER 3

IN THE BEGINNING

WUHAN

Nestled in the interior of China some 500 miles west of Shanghai is a large city called Wuhan in the Hubei Province, the largest city not on China's east coast. Around 11,000,000 people live in Wuhan, making it bigger than New York City. It's the capital of all things central China – transportation, commerce, education, finance, culture, perhaps most analogous to Chicago in the United States.

The Yangtze River slices through Wuhan on its meandering way east to Shanghai and the Pacific Ocean. Wuhan is largely a manufacturing-oriented city. Tall glass buildings, advanced industries, mass transit, five levels of expressways crisscrossing -- this is no small town lost in time.

Dongfeng Motor Group is headquartered there, a $9.4B corporation employing nearly 150,000 people (not all in Wuhan). General Motors and affiliated partners employ 6,000 people in Wuhan. Nissan and Honda also have a large presence there. Over 500 car parts manufacturers operate in Wuhan, making it the largest industry in the city. Apple produces iPhones in the Hubei Province. Most major American fast food chains have a presence there. PepsiCo and Siemens have large operations there.

Wuhan sports downtown skyscrapers, riverboats, restaurants and more street food vendors than everything in America combined. Hubu Alley is a local and tourist must-visit destination in Wuhan. It is comparable to the Grand and Spice Bazaar in Istanbul or the Wharf in San Francisco, densely filled with local food vendors for nearly the length of two football fields. Comparing it to the Seattle fish market would not do it justice. Activity favorites in Wuhan include plays, musicals and opera, food exploration, water sports and fishing and shopping, much like all large metropolitan areas.

Like many Chinese cities, Wuhan also boasts something you don't see in most western cities or in much of America: wet markets. Many foods may be found in these wet markets. Three-year aged ham, raw chickens in open air, vegetables of all varieties, fish, things you may see in Chinatown in New York or San Francisco. What won't you see in Chinatown in New York or San Francisco that you may have seen in Wuhan's wet markets? There are live exotic and domestic animals traded. In street shops you may see a hanging dead porcupine, badgers, bamboo rats, snakes, bats and civets.

Sometime in November of 2019, a new (novel) virus to be called SARS-CoV-2 infected victim one, according to the *South Morning China Post*. Coronavirus disease 2019 (COVID-19) is caused by severe acute respiratory syndrome coronavirus 2 (SARS-CoV-2). Consensus is it began in Wuhan. Consensus also says it was sourced from a bat; it has a 96% whole-genome overlap with a coronavirus found in bats. Beyond that there is much speculation. Some believe an infected Chinese horseshoe bat passed it on to another animal that passed it on to a human. Horseshoe bats are not common to Wuhan; they are native hundreds of miles away.

That intermediary animal may have been a cat, cow, civet, or dromedary camel passed in similar fashion to how the 2002 SARS outbreak was passed along. A popular suspect is the pangolin, a scaly anteater-looking animal prized for its meat and the medicinal properties of its scales. Have you seen one? Almost prehistoric looking.

Professor Robert Webster published a great white paper in 2004 on wet markets and the threat they pose to spreading SARS coronaviruses.[10] Webster wrote of how SARS and the H5N1 bird flu virus originated in Chinese wet markets and predicted a SARS coronavirus would originate there and become threatening. Animals that could pass it on may be red-meat market civets or raccoon dogs.

In the United States, there are live poultry markets that have been associated with flu viruses H5 and H7; they threaten commercial poultry production. Those H5 and H7 viruses had not moved from animals to humans in America. While wet markets aren't commonplace in the U.S., in New York the number of live poultry markets nearly doubled to 80 in New York City in the early 2000's. Civet cats were once banned in Chinese wet markets but came back. They sold for about $200, but not as pets.

Webster went on to warn that beyond wet markets, laboratories could be a source of SARS coronavirus spreads. He cited two cases of that very thing happening, in Singapore and in Taiwan. He also said the reemergence of H1N1 viruses came back in the 1970's from a laboratory. He predicted a pandemic outbreak was a real threat from the wet markets and from China.

Another theory swirling around is that the coronavirus came from a bat but was exposed to someone from the Wuhan Institute of Virology in Wuhan. The Wuhan Institute houses the largest virus bank in Asia which preserves more than 1,500 strains.[11] The United States cited this laboratory with a safety violation warning in 2019, but many labs have the potential for leaks, as Professor Webster cited. An American laboratory accidentally shipped live anthrax to the American base in South Korea and several labs in the states in 2015.

CASE ONE

The first COVID-19 case reported was a 57-year-old woman feeling flu-like symptoms and admitting herself to a clinic on December 10, 2019. Within days she found herself ill and not responsive to anti-flu remedies. Following the first case, a handful of cases were reported each day with the cases grown to sixty by December 20, 2019.

Dr. Ai Fen was the head of the Wuhan Central Hospital at the time. She was reviewing data of the patients with respiratory symptoms that were not improving. When Ai reviewed lab results of one of the cases on December 30, 2019, she was shocked to learn of a presence of a SARS coronavirus. She circulated that information within her healthcare circle.

WHISTLEBLOWER

Li Wenliang was a 34-year-old ophthalmologist practicing in Wuhan and was one of the doctors that got wind of Ai Fen's findings. On December 30, he sent a note to peer doctors suggesting they exercise extra care and that there was an outbreak of a SARS-type illness. Hospital or healthcare leadership instructed Fen to keep it quiet to avoid a panic. The Public Security Bureau in Wuhan reached out to Wenliang and made him sign a statement renouncing his days-earlier findings. Wenliang is considered a true whistleblower for coming out with the information knowing of potential consequences from the Chinese government.

Wenliang caught the virus from a glaucoma patient positive with it on January 8. The patient worked at a store in the seafood market in Wuhan. Reports are that Wenliang felt ill within two days, spent the next couple weeks in intensive care and was quarantined while it was confirmed he was positive for the virus.

By all accounts, Wenliang was healthy, obviously young and his demographic was not typically at serious risk. That proved not to be the case, perhaps because his patient from whom he caught the virus had a high load ratio. Wenliang died on February 7, 2020 and should be remembered for bravery and courage for speaking out, knowing the possible consequences within his home country.

WUHAN'S OUTBREAK

The Lancet published a study in January analyzing the first Wuhan infected patients.[12] A majority of the initial patients had contact with the Huanan Seafood Wholesale Market in Wuhan, and the first patient known to die had repeated contact there. He was admitted to the hospital with traditional flu-like symptoms and worsening respiratory symptoms. Based on analysis of the initial cases, the timeline for those symptomatic and infected looked something like this:

1. Day one – infection
2. Day seven – admission to hospital with flu-like and respiratory issues
3. Day ten – admission to an intensive care unit
4. Day fourteen – removal from intensive care unit, or death

This timeline has largely held as infections spread across the world. We later learned that if you contracted it and were going to be symptomatic, symptoms would occur quickly.

By January 2, 2020, 41 people in Wuhan were admitted to the hospital with COVID-19. Any of the data that has come out of China is not necessarily reliable, as none of this has been transparent. Quoting *The Lancet* report:

*   *Most of the infected patients were men (30 [73%] of 41)*
*   *Less than half had underlying diseases (13 [32%]), including diabetes (eight [20%]), hypertension (six [15%]), and cardiovascular disease (six [15%])*
*   *Median age was 49 years*
*   *27 (66%) of 41 patients had been exposed to Huanan seafood market. One family cluster was found.*
*   *Common symptoms at onset of illness were fever (40 [98%] of 41 patients), cough (31 [76%]), and myalgia or fatigue (18 [44%])*

- *Less common symptoms were sputum production (11 [28%] of 39), headache (three [8%] of 38), haemoptysis (two [5%] of 39), and yspnea (one [3%] of 38). Dyspnoea developed in 22 (55%) of 40 patients (median time from illness onset to yspnea 8·0 days [IQR 5·0–13·0]). 26 (63%) of 41 patients had lymphopenia*
- *All 41 patients had pneumonia with abnormal findings on chest CT.*
- *Complications included acute respiratory distress syndrome (12 [29%]), RNAaemia (six [15%]), acute cardiac injury (five [12%]) and secondary infection (four [10%]). 13 (32%) patients were admitted to an ICU and six (15%) died*

On March 9, 2020, *The Lancet* published a study based on the first 191 patients from two hospitals in Wuhan titled, *Clinical course and risk factors for mortality of adult inpatients with COVID-19 in Wuhan, China: a retrospective cohort study.* Of the 191 patients included in the study, 137 survived the virus and 54 did not. Below are some excerpts from the study:

- *67% of the non-survivors had a comorbidity condition, meaning the presence of more than one chronic condition, such as hypertension, coronary heart disease or diabetes*
- *The study includes 29 of the original 41 diagnosed with COVID-19 (named for corona virus disease 2019)*
- *Average age of the non-survivors was 69 years old (ranging 63 years old to 76 years old)*
- *39/54 non-survivors were men*

This report is incredibly detailed and was available prior to the lockdown measures taken across the world in later March. More on that later.

CHINA ACTIONS

On January 23, 2020, China shut down several cities to contain the spread of COVID-19, including Wuhan, Zhijiang (about 200 miles from Wuhan), Chibi, Exhou and Huanggang. All in about fifty million people were under lockdown. This would go on for more than two months. At the time that seemed unfathomable.

No one imagined then that billions would be locked down within weeks worldwide. By this time, cases had been discovered in the United States, Singapore, Hong Kong, the United Kingdom, South Korea, Japan and Thailand.

Travel outside of those Chinese cities was out, whether by train, plane, ferries or any mass transit. Movie theaters, restaurants and non-necessary businesses were shut down. At this time, according to Chinese releases, under a thousand cases were confirmed, under a hundred people were hospitalized and about twenty-five had died.

By January 24, grocery store shelves emptied as people stocked up. Subway stations were chained shut. Everyone wore masks. The streets were quiet. Online shopping took off at Taobao, China's largest ecommerce company. In late January, as Americans watched the news of China's lockdown, it's unthinkable that anyone saw these lockdowns coming to America just weeks later. Through early data from the Chinese, it was already known by an albeit small sampling that the fatalities come from an identifiable segment of the population.

ITALY

On January 30, 2019, Italian Prime Minister Giuseppe Conte stated there were two confirmed cases of COVID-19 in Italy. By the end of January, Italy ceased all flights from China, Hong Kong and Taiwan. We would later see Italy with the first and one of the highest outbreaks in Europe, along with many questions about why that occurred.

Italy's population is just over 60,000,000 people and life expectancy is 84 years old. Around 23% of the population is considered aging (over 65 years old), and 13% under 15, illustrating an aging population mix.

The Lombardy region is home to ten million residents including its capital city, Milan. The Emilia-Romagna region, adjacent south to the Lombardy region, is home to 4.4 million people. Both are considered northern Italy. They mirror the age demographics of the country.

Going back to 2019, Italy was the second most struggling country economically behind only Greece in the European Union. Italy has struggled since the 2008 financial crisis and has been hit harder than most EU countries with unplanned and uncontrolled immigration from North Africa, mostly refugees from Libya, and domestic economic challenges. In 2018, Italy had negative GDP growth for two consecutive quarters to finish off the year, officially placing it in a recession.

While the United States was very healthy economically, some countries in the EU were struggling. Italy has the fourth largest economy in the EU (behind Germany, UK and France). Feeling left behind and struggling with the EU leadership in Brussels over options, they entered into a partnership with China.

IRAN

Iran has a population of nearly 84,000,000. Incredibly, only 5.5% of the population is over 65 years old.[13] Iran's economy is driven by the oil and gas industries and a dominant part of government revenue is exporting fossil fuel products. Iran ranks within the top four countries worldwide in natural gas and crude oil reserves. Iran's currency dipped fourfold in currency trade compared to the U.S. dollar in 2019.

In 2018, inflation reached 40%--think hard about that. Unemployment reached 12% (just below what the United States saw during the lockdowns). Their economy shrunk for two straight years and the U.S. renewed sanctions following the pullout of the Iran Nuclear Deal, choking their economy. The U.S. imposed sanctions on any country that traded with Iran, impacting the large oil and gas exports and the second largest export industry of Iran, steel and mining.

ONE BELT ONE ROAD

In the first half of 2019, struggling with their economies, Iran and Italy both signed an agreement with China called the One Belt One Road (OBOR) initiative. The Belt and Road initiative was a project Chinese President Xi Jinping began in 2013. The purpose is to strengthen trade and infrastructure development between China and other countries. Conceptually, the "belt" was to mirror old silk trade routes of the past, and the "road" was to open shipping trade.

Simply put, a country enters into the agreement with China. They agree on projects or trade deals. Financing is provided by China, as well as products and labor if the projects were infrastructure-related. Over a hundred countries signed on by 2019. The Chinese motivation is obvious: get other countries indebted to China and create jobs and revenues for China.

The relevance to this is that Iran and Italy were the hardest hit initial countries outside China for COVID-19. It is possible their close connections to China enabled the quick spread.

Helen Raleigh wrote an interesting article for *The Federalist* on March 17, 2020.[14] She made a strong case for outlining how the One Belt One Road agreements between Italy-China and Iran-China were the differentiating factors in those two countries experiencing some of the first and highest impacts of COVID-19. Both are geographically far and remote from China, the center of the outbreak.

With a weak economy, Italy entered into the agreement a year before the outbreak, the largest EU country to join. Raleigh wrote:

> *"Lombardy and Tuscany are the two regions that saw the most Chinese investment. Nearly a year later, the first Wuhan coronavirus infection case in Italy was reported in the Lombardy region on Feb. 21. Today, Italy is experiencing the worst coronavirus outbreak outside China, and Lombardy is the hardest-hit region in the country."*

Iran joined the China agreement just after Italy. Raleigh did an excellent job outlining the connection between One Belt One Road and the severe breakout in Iran:

> *"Facing domestic economic and political challenges and international isolation, Iran has sought out China as an ally against the United States, relying on economic ties and military cooperation with Beijing to fend off U.S.-imposed sanctions. China has been keeping the Iranian regime afloat by purchasing Iranian oil, selling the Iranian regime weapons, and transferring nuclear technologies.*

> *"But 2019 was the year Iran officially signed up to OBOR. China sees Iran as a crucial player to this initiative because Iran is not only rich in oil but also lies in a direct path of an ambitious 2,000-mile railroad China wants to build, which will run from western China through Tehran and Turkey into Europe.*

> *"Today, Iranian health officials trace the country's coronavirus outbreak to Qom, a city of a million people. According to the Wall Street Journal, "China Railway Engineering Corp. is building a $2.7 billion high-speed rail line through Qom. Chinese technicians have been helping refurbish a nuclear-power plant nearby." Iranian medical professionals suspect either Chinese workers in Qom or an Iranian businessman who travelled to China from Qom caused the spread of the coronavirus in Qom."*

JANUARY TIMELINE

Looking back at the timeline in January, we can see the wildfire-like spread of information and actions taken worldwide.

December 31, 2019: Wuhan Municipal Health reports unusual cases of pneumonia discovered that month in Wuhan, no virus identified.

January 1, 2020: Huanan Seafood Wholesale Market closes when it's considered exotic animals traded there may be the source of the illnesses.

January 7, 2020: China identifies novel (new strain) coronavirus as the source of the new illnesses.

January 11, 2020: 61-year-old man is first to die from COVID-19.

January 13, 2020: First case outside China is identified in Thailand from a Chinese national traveling from Wuhan.

January 16, 2020: Japanese man identified with virus in Japan after traveling to China.

January 17, 2020: The United States began testing travelers for symptoms at airports in San Francisco, New York and Los Angeles.

January 21, 2020: First United States citizen known to be infected in Washington state.

January 29, 2020: American Airlines announces it will suspend flights between major U.S. and China cities beginning February 9, 2020.

January 30, 2020: The Allied Pilots Association, which represents American Airlines' 15,000 pilots, sued AA on Thursday to stop the carrier from flying to China and filed an injunction to halt the flights to and from China immediately.

January 31, 2020: President Trump announces the United States will deny entrance to America of any travelers from China within the previous 14 days. For Americans returning home from there they would be quarantined; the Pentagon said it would provide housing for 1,000 people until February 29.

EXPERT OPINIONS AT THE TIME

When January was winding down, most impacts of COVID-19 were unclear. At the time, President Trump's clamp on entrance to the United States from China was harshly criticized by his critics in the media and his political opposition. It was a bold move and other countries like Australia echoed the move. Critics saw it as a way for him to hurt China given the years of trade negotiations and disdain he exhibited for the U.S.-China trade deficit, lost manufacturing jobs and Chinese theft of intellectual property.

The World Health Organization made a comment on January 31, 2020:

> *"Travel restrictions can cause more harm than good by hindering info-sharing, medical supply chains and harming economies," the head of the World Health Organization (WHO) said on Friday. "The WHO recommends introducing screening at official border crossings. It has warned that closing borders could accelerate the spread of the virus, with travelers entering countries unofficially. "Just as the WHO recommended against travel restrictions, the U.S. rushed in the opposite direction," foreign ministry spokeswoman Hua Chunying said. "[It is] certainly not a gesture of goodwill."*[15]

On what planet can closing borders accelerate the spread of anything? And, if your mission is health care and pandemic prevention, how much should a "gesture of goodwill" even factor in? This isn't an ethical debate. This was a genuine policy move aimed at slowing down the spread of a foreign virus.

CNN reported about the travel ban on February 7, 2020.[16] Writer Catherine Shoichet's premise is that a travel ban can hurt more than help a spreading pandemic. You be the judge and keep this in mind: a travel ban objective is to stop or slow the spread of something from one host country to another, something spread person-to-person.

> *"With this virus, like others that have come before it, one key tool investigators have as they try to treat it and stop it from spreading is the information individuals share about their symptoms and behavior," the report said. "And a travel ban can get in the way of that, public health experts say."*

So, a temporary travel ban with China will discourage infected and symptomatic people from speaking out about their symptoms? But the travel ban prevents, in theory, infected and non-infected travelers from reaching another country anyway, so isn't their candor moot? The reporting continued:

> *"On a personal level, it discourages people from coming forward, from being transparent," says Saskia Popescu, an epidemiologist in Arizona and global health security researcher at George Mason University. "You're more likely to have people try and go about travel in less direct ways, which would then totally negate the purpose of that. You're forcing people into situations that could more actively promote disease transmission."*

On this premise, the suggestion is that infected people may be forced into situations that more actively promote SARS transmission. From another continent with an ocean between it and America?

> *One reason countries may be wary of sharing information: the economic consequences of a travel ban can be devastating.*
>
> *"It has massive economic implications," Popescu says.*
>
> *Eric Carter, an associate professor of geography and global health at Macalaster College who studies the politics of public health, points to what happened in West Africa during the Ebola outbreak as an example.*
>
> *"First of all, it made it harder to some degree for health personnel to get into the country, to actually do the work they needed to do," he says. "Also, it just so severely damaged the economies of those western African countries that were affected by Ebola, because they were cut off from the rest of the world. Other countries weren't even buying what they produced. That ended up having really dramatic effects."*
>
> *The latest U.S. restrictions could stop hundreds of thousands of people from visiting the United States each month and "come with huge economic and societal impacts," says Sarah Pierce, a policy analyst at the Migration Policy Institute in Washington.*
>
> *"The way it's written, it seems like it's going to be impossible for Chinese nationals to be granted visas," she told CNN. "This is a massive flow that*

this ban is restricting with very little evidence that it's actually going to benefit the United States."

To be fair to everyone cited in this article, no one at this time saw the worldwide lockdowns coming just six weeks from this publication. To also be fair, CNN is predominantly contrarian to any President Trump policy. President Trump executed a travel ban to slow down what most think may be a pandemic coming from China.

In April, as President Trump is championing opening America up, CNN spent much of their analysis debunking that approach until a plurality of Americans could be tested for SARS-CoV-2 (or until the election). CNN's February report continued:

World Health Organization Director-General Tedros Adhanom Ghebreyesus warned this week that travel bans might do more harm than good.

"Such restrictions can have the effect of increasing fear and stigma, with little public health benefit," he said Tuesday in Geneva. "Where such measures have been implemented, we urge that they are short in duration, proportionate to the public health risks, and are reconsidered regularly as the situation evolves."

Carter told CNN the past provides plenty of examples of travel restrictions stigmatizing countries and ethnicities. The response to the novel coronavirus, including recent travel restrictions, has happened more quickly than in past epidemics -- and from a public health standpoint, that could be a good thing, he says. But he notes there are also other questions to consider.

"Historically a lot of these border security measures have used public health as a pretext for discrimination. It's very easy to see how a public health rationale would be used to limit immigration for whatever reason," he says. "And I'm not saying that that's actually occurring, but it well could in this particular political climate, not just in the US, but internationally."

Read the part above once more, and then consider this was published with no counter opinion. A representative from the WHO, *the* world health organization, is concerned about fear and stigma. At this time, there is credible reason to fear a virus that unquestionably launched out of Wuhan. You have a few thousand people infected in China. It's a big enough deal that China locked their cities down.

You don't want it to spread into America until it gets figured out, so you stop travel between there and America. This was not just conjecture; two weeks before this article was published, China locked down its own cities. It's poor journalism to not represent balance. It's an implausible argument to fault the government from winding down flights to and from a place that has locked down its own people for fear of spreading.

MEDIA COVERAGE

The media downplayed and largely dismissed the threat of the coronavirus in America in January 2020.

On January 25, Dr. John Torres, NBC News Medical Correspondent, said *"You're hearing a lot of news about [COVID-19] right now, but the reality is comparing it to the flu, it's not even close to that stage."* The point here is that a subject matter expert like Torres did not see this coming.

On January 31, Dr. Sanjay Gupta was on CNN interviewed by Alisyn Camerota and she said *"…there's an important context we need to keep this in, that the flu is more deadly [than COVID-19],"* to which he replied, *"This is one of the ironies that keeps coming up. Take a look at the numbers."* He was referencing the number of flu deaths compared to COVID-19. However, it's easy to see news-opinion people and a subject matter expert not seeing the eventual impact COVID-19 would have on the United States and the world. (source: CNN broadcast)

On February 1, 2020, former vice president Joe Biden tweeted this on Twitter in response to the halt on China travelers to America:

> *"We are in the midst of a crisis with the coronavirus. We need to lead the way with science — not Donald Trump's record of hysteria, xenophobia, and fearmongering. He is the worst possible person to lead our country through a global health emergency."* [17]

Looking back, it is hard to view the policy as xenophobic. Mr. Biden?

INTERNATIONAL REACTION

As you see the timeline unfold, the first COVID-19 death was on January 11,

2020. Just twenty days later, at the end of January, with fewer than fifty total deaths, it's incredible to look back at the swiftness of how many countries took action. By the end of January:

- Hong Kong banned any travelers from Hubei Province (the province Wuhan resides).
- Iran suspended all flights to and from China.
- Italy suspended all flights to and from China, Hong Kong and Taiwan.
- Laos closed its border with China.
- Sri-Lanka, Malaysia suspended visas-on-arrival to Chinese nationals from Hubei Province.
- Afghanistan closed its border with China.
- The Bahamas did not allow any non-citizen to enter the Bahamas if they had been to China in the last twenty days.
- Singapore suspended new and existing visas from China nationals and suspended entrance of any foreign national if they'd been to China within fourteen days.
- Russia closed its border with China.
- Philippines suspended visa-free travel from China.
- North Korea closed its borders with Russia and China, as well as entrance to North Korea if one of their citizens or a foreign national had been to China and suspended all flights to China.
- Guatemala banned anyone who had been to China within the previous fifteen days.

THE UNITED STATES ECONOMY

These headlines tell you a lot about the state of the economy as 2020 was beginning:

Unemployment was holding strong in January 2020 hovering around the 50-year low of 3.6%[18]

Colorado unemployment rate reaches historic low of 2.5%; State's tight labor market enters a third year[19]

Utah's unemployment rate is now at an all-time low[20]

US weekly jobless claims increase less than expected[21]

Florida's unemployment rate hits record low[22]

New jobless claims fall 5th straight week to 204,000 in sign of strong U.S. labor market[23]

Washington state unemployment rate hits new low[24]

Michigan's seasonally adjusted unemployment rate crept down one-tenth of a percentage point to 3.9 percent last month with payroll jobs increasing by 5,000 in December[25]

California unemployment holds at record low 3.9 percent in December; Employers add 12,600 nonfarm jobs as record job expansion continues[26]

Dow Jones Industrial Average closes above 29,000 for first time[27]

Rank-and-File Workers Get Bigger Raises; Short supply of labor, minimum-wage rises and increased poaching have helped lift wages for lower-income workers. [28]

The Wall Street Journal article above went on to say,

"Wages for rank-and-file workers are rising at the quickest pace in more than a decade, even faster than for bosses, a sign that the labor market has tightened sufficiently to convey bigger increases to lower-paid employees. Gains for those workers have accelerated much of this year, a time when the unemployment rate fell to a half-century low. A short supply of workers, increased poaching and minimum-wage increases have helped those nearer to the bottom of the pay scale."

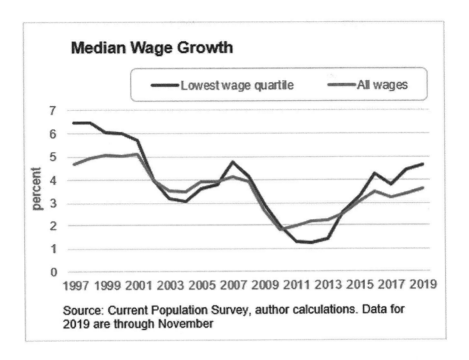

Median Wage Growth

Source: Current Population Survey, author calculations. Data for 2019 are through November

The chart above published by the Federal Reserve of Atlanta reflecting data through November 2019 illustrates higher wage growth for lower income workers than higher income workers. The top line is the lowest wage quartile and the lower line is all wages. By any real measure within the past fifty years, when considering record low unemployment, wage growth and the all-time high of The Dow Jones Industrial Average (DJIA) index, the economy was about as strong as possible. By the end of January, COVID-19 was catching frequent attention by the media and political leaders. Even then no one saw how the next ninety days would unfold.

If you follow President Trump and his economic messages, and a data point he looks at in reflecting the health of the economy, it's the stock market indexes. When Trump was inaugurated in 2017, the DJIA was 19,827.25. It peaked well over 29,000 in February 2020 before the threat of the economic impact of COVID-19 began.

Pundits debate the value of the index as a reflection of the economy. Critics say it reflects the wealthy and that most people don't own stocks. That's not really the point. The market index reflects the valuation of stocks that comprise it. If those stocks are up, the companies inside it are either doing great or expected to do great. Stocks rise based on current performance or a positive outlook. In January 2020 the outlook was as bright as we'd seen in decades.

CHAPTER 4

OUTBREAK

FEBRUARY 2020

On February 1, Americans were waking up to headlines that flights to and from China had been cancelled. Still, most Americans were not thinking about SARS-CoV-2. The Super Bowl was the evening of February 2, and Kansas City fans were going to finally find peace of mind. The sports world was still reeling from Kobe Bryant's untimely passing. The Democrats were beginning the process of selecting their presidential nominee and that was consuming news. Socialist populist Bernie Sanders was looking like the sure bet to win that nomination and challenge Donald Trump for the presidency in November.

Back in Wuhan, Li Wenliang was struggling in intensive care and would not survive to week two. Wuhan was entering the second week of their lockdown and most westerners felt this was a China epidemic and it was just a headline. Then word spread of a cruise ship infected with COVID-19 off the coast of Japan. The Diamond Princess cruise ship was informed of a disembarked passenger with the virus. Days later the cruise was cancelled and the ship was quarantined in Japan while testing each passenger and crew took place.

Many countries ceased flights to and from China, Taiwan and Hong Kong. Still, it was viewed at the time as more preventive than anything. On February 3, *The New York Times* ran an article with this sub-headline: "The C.D.C. is testing three patients in the city for coronavirus. Should New Yorkers be worried, and what could happen next?"[29] What indeed. No one imagined what would unfold in New York in mere weeks and then last for months.

Further in that article was this:

Public health officials note that the ordinary flu has proved to be far more dangerous so far. Across the country, the C.D.C. says 68 children have died of the flu this year, and the agency estimates 10,000 adults have died. The coronavirus has not yet caused a single death in the United States, officials said. At a news conference, Mayor Bill de Blasio said transmission of the new coronavirus required "substantial contact with someone who already has it," adding that "you don't get it" from touching a surface.

This is no indictment of the *Times* or the mayor. It simply was not viewed as a threat at the time.

DR. ANTHONY FAUCI

Dr. Anthony Fauci is the director of the National Institute of Allergy and Infectious Diseases at the National Institutes of Health for the federal government. Dr. Fauci reached worldwide prominence in just weeks by providing daily updates with President Trump, Vice President Pence and other medical experts including Deborah Birx, a physician specializing in HIV/AIDS immunology and vaccine research.

Here are some comments Fauci made on CBS Face The Nation on February 16, 2020:

"A pandemic is when you have multiple countries throughout the world that have what's called sustained transmission from person to person to person, multiple generations. Right now, there are 24 countries in which there were over five hundred cases. Several of them are starting to get to the second and third transmission. So technically speaking, the WHO wouldn't be calling this a global pandemic, but it certainly is on the verge of that happening reasonably soon unless containment is more successful than it is right now.

"This virus, we don't know. But it is not unreasonable to say that influenza, for example, which peaks in the winter, you would certainly expect it by March, April and May to taper down, as well as typical common cold coronaviruses. That's not an unreasonable statement. However, we do not know what this particular virus is gonna do so. So we would think it would be a stretch to assume that it's going to disappear with the warm weather. We don't know that. It's completely unknown."[30]

The coronavirus was more a headline in February than anything causing change in America, until American-Chinese supply chains began to fracture and the stock market crashed at the end of the month. In Europe, the wave was beginning to reach the border of many countries.

FIRST COVID-19 FATALITIES

COUNTRY	FIRST COVID-19 FATALITY
China	1/10/2020
United States	2/06/2020
Japan	2/12/2020
France	2/15/2020
Iran	2/18/2020
Italy	2/22/2020
Australia	2/29/2020
Sweden	3/10/2020
Spain	3/2/2020
United Kingdom	3/5/2020
Germany	3/8/2020

The first major international headline outside Wuhan came on February 5, when the Diamond Princess cruise ship was quarantined with cases identified. The World Health Organization named the disease sourced from SARS-CoV-2 and called it COVID-19.

The New York Times reported on February 24, "the Trump administration, after weeks of pleading from lawmakers, asked Congress on Monday to allocate $1.25 billion in new emergency funds to bolster its coronavirus response." The funds would be spent on "medical research and supplies" in preparation for what might come.[31]

TRAVEL

By the end of February, the following countries had travel bans to and from China:[32]

Australia - Any foreign nationals in mainland China will not be allowed to enter Australia until 14 days after they have left or transited through China. Australian citizens, permanent residents and their families are able to enter but must isolate themselves for 14 days if they've recently been to mainland China. The government has advised against any travel to mainland China.

Hong Kong – Quarantine required for anyone arriving from mainland China, including Hong Kong residents and visitors beginning February 8.

India - Existing visas are no longer valid for any foreign national traveling from China and anyone traveling from China will be quarantined.

Japan – Foreign nationals who have visited China's Hubei province denied entry into Japan, and these limitations would be expanded.

New Zealand - Banned anyone traveling from China on February 3.

Philippines - Banned visitors from China, Hong Kong and Macau. Any Philippine returning from China would be quarantined.

Saudi Arabia - citizens banned travel to China and those trying to return would not be allowed.

South Korea – no foreigners allowed entry that had visited or stayed in Hubei in the previous 14 days.

Italy – banned travel to and from China and entry from those coming from China on February 27. Italy would lock down many towns on February 23.

United States – implemented restricted travel to and from China, Iran, Italy and South Korea.

Also, companies around the globe began to stop business travel. For example, in February, Nestle stopped or severely limited international business travel for its nearly 300,000 employees. British American Tobacco Plc, Coca-Cola, Kraft Heinz Co. acted similarly. At this point, France had not cancelled their spring fashion shows, that would change soon. Amazon limited employee travel and Apple stopped employee travel to China except for emergency purposes, same for Facebook and Google. Microsoft instructed employees in China to work from home.

ECONOMICS

MANUFACTURING

CNBC reported in mid-February that up to five million companies have touches of operations in China that would be affected.[33] How? Dun and Bradstreet wrote that 15% of the Fortune 1000 companies have operations that would be interrupted by the initial Chinese quarantines. Though the direct impact was not yet felt in America, two major economic impacts began.

First, many companies sell products that are made in China. If they aren't producing or there is a halt on shipping from China, companies don't have products to sell. Second, China is the second largest consumer of products. If they are locked down, they aren't spending money on American-produced or other-made products. Companies like General Motors, Ford Motor Tesla, have significant operations in China that would halt manufacturing.

China manufactures all or a dominant amount of many industrial and household products that are economic and "life-essential."[34]

China exports the highest value of computer sales and just over 40% of all computer sales worldwide. China is not just a huge consumer of cell phones, they make them. Huawei Technologies, Apple, Guangdong Oppo Mobile, Vivo Communication Technology, Xiaomi Technology, and until last year, Samsung, all manufactured cell phones in China. Nike, Adidas, and many other shoe companies have a high percentage of their products manufactured in China. On top of manufacturing Nike closed about half their stores in China.

SERVICE INDUSTRIES AND RETAIL

Ten to twenty percent of McDonald's restaurants in China (more than 3,000) closed in February. Yum Brands, the operator of the KFC and Pizza Hut franchises in China, said nearly one-third of its restaurants closed because of the outbreak. The remaining stores saw a major drop in sales.

Starbucks closed more than half of its 4,300 stores in China and delayed a planned update to its 2020 financial forecast, saying it expects a large but temporary hit.

This doesn't even touch the huge impact Chinese companies servicing residents felt. It will mirror the April impact in the United States.

Below is a chart that illustrates back in February 2020 the forecasted downturn industries projected from China's lockdown and interrupted supply chain alone:

1Q end product shipment in millions:[35]

1Q 2020	PREVIOUS FORECAST	REVISED FORECAST	% CHANGE
Smart Watches	14.4	12.1	-16.0%
Smartphones	307	275	-10.4%
Notebooks	35	30.7	-12.3%
Monitors	29	27.5	-5.2%
TVs	48.8	46.6	-4.5%
Video Game Consoles	6.9	6.2	-10.1%
Smart Speakers	26.4	23.2	-12.1%
Automobiles	21	19.3	-8.1%

By the end of February, the United States was not impacted in a lifestyle way or with illnesses, but the stock market began reeling. Remember, even though the United States was not yet feeling the pain, companies were. Forecasts were down for many products as illustrated by TrendForce above. Travel was down, so airline and any hospitality industry-related companies (hotels, for example), were seeing drastic revenue decreases.

Companies like Apple lost manufacturing and supply chain production, so they had less to sell. Also, the huge consumer market in China was now suppressed. If sales projections drop for so many corporations, their earnings would drop year over year. Investors would consider them devalued and then reinvest from these companies, putting their money in less vulnerable industries or companies affected by these market and supply chain compromises.

INVESTOR IMPACTS

By the end of February, the U.S. stock market indexes suffered their worst week since the financial collapse twelve years earlier. The Dow Jones Industrial Average lost nearly 20% of its value in one week. Most 401K investors hold various kinds of funds, weighting their risk amongst many stocks. They suffered huge decreases in value. When President Trump reached office in 2017, the DJIA was under 20,000, and in the first quarter 2020 climbed to over 29,000.

American Airlines lost a full third of their stock value in just three weeks. Carnival Corporation lost over a third, Delta Airlines dropped a quarter. Apple Corporation, one of the highest valued companies in the world, shed 15% of its value in ten days. The unemployment rate in the United States was still a healthy 3.6%, but that was about to change too.

CHAPTER 5

THE CRUISE SHIPS

It's the mid-1980s. Many questions are swirling about HIV. Health experts, scientists and governments around the world are all curious to learn about the spread of the virus. Dr. Fauci himself speculated in 1983 that HIV could be transmitted by skin-to-skin touch.[36] They know it's predominately sexually transmitted. Nearly all cases at this time are between gay men, and curiosity is piqued around its ease of spread, spread within heterosexuals, and any other ways it can get from person to person.

They decide to set up a scientific experiment. They recruit 2,000 single swingers to go on a cruise for three weeks. They choose an even balance of men and women, encourage bisexual passengers, and people of all races age 18-80. The crew staff of 500 is not allowed to have any sexual contact with the passengers. The cruise will be at sea for the twenty-one days. At the end of the cruise they interview each passenger and trace everyone's contact, whether sexual, hand-to-hand social contact, who participated in what, and then test everyone when they port in and for the next twelve months.

Can you imagine a better scientific experiment? A large controlled environment, limited variables, it's the optimum petri dish for testing virus spread among people. No, this didn't actually happen, but it did happen by accident more than once in February 2020. Incredible insight into the spread of the SARS-CoV-2 was gained. However, little of the analytics were factored into the policy decisions leaders made and the media encouraged in March 2020.

THE DIAMOND PRINCESS

The Diamond Princess cruise ship first launched in 2004 by the Carnival Corporation. Carnival owns multiple cruise lines. Princess was made famous by the television show, *The Love Boat*, back in the 1970's and 1980's. The Diamond Princess accommodates 2,670 passengers and is supported by 1,100 crew members. It's a city on the sea if you've ever been. Countless dining opportunities, a casino, live entertainment, multiple pools, sports activities, and interesting places to visit on the port days.

On January 20, 2019, the Diamond Princess left Yokohama, Japan at full capacity for a fourteen-day cruise. Passengers were surely excited to visit ports in China, Vietnam and Taiwan. On January 27, a passenger left the cruise ship in Hong Kong. That passenger was diagnosed with COVID-19 on February 1. By February 4, the cruise itinerary was cancelled. On that day, 10 people positive for COVID-19 were released for medical care, and by February 6, 41 people tested positive. What ensued was a near month-long quarantine.

Many in the media and medical community criticized the cruise ship quarantine. Unfairly. If you imagine being in the decision-making capacity, there are limited choices. Data was not really known about the ability to spread and the lethality of the virus. At this point, it was new to the world for thirty days and not yet really impacted anywhere outside China. As many in the world sat locked down in their own homes from March to June 2020, pause for a moment to imagine being quarantined on a cruise ship.

Nearly all the rooms are small. Many have balconies but more do not. The casino is now closed. Live group entertainment is cancelled. You know some portion of the people with whom you are seeing and interacting have the new virus. You don't really know how contagious or dangerous it is, but the actions taken are extreme and you've seen *Outbreak* and *Contagion*. If there's a moment a situation seems unbearable, other than prison it's hard to imagine something more difficult than those days. Not just the confinement but the uncertainty of what will happen.

The Center for Mathematical Modeling for Infectious Diseases performed a very detailed study of the Diamond Princess passenger demographics, published on March 23, 2020.[37] Over the page is the make-up of the passengers:

AGE	PASSENGERS	COVID-19 POSITIVE W/SYMPTOMS	COVID-19 POSITIVE W/NO SYMPTOMS
0 - 9	16	0	1
10-19	23	2	3
20 - 29	347	25	3
30 - 39	428	27	7

40 - 49	334	19	8
50 - 59	398	28	31
60 - 69	923	76	101
70 - 79	1015	95	139
80 - 89	216	29	25
Totals	**3700**	**301**	**318**

The passengers and crew gave the world an unexpected gift of data about COVID-19. It was the best possible [accidental] controlled experiment a scientist could hope for to study the spread and impact of anything. From that cruise we see 3,700 people on board, and a quarter for certain caught COVID-19 or were carrying SARS-CoV-2.

Half were asymptomatic. Seven elderly passengers died from it. Of those seven, two were an elderly Japanese couple in their 80's with underlying conditions.[38] It's very sad to see that a couple enjoying an elaborate vacation would not survive it due to this unforeseen occurrence. The other five passengers that did not survive were all over 70 as well.

While this was one excellent data point, it offered up that COVID-19 is threatening to the elderly and, moreover, those with an underlying respiratory condition.

The Lancet is one of the best known and relied upon medical journal repositories, founded in 1823 by Thomas Wakley. They have published over 10,000 articles since inception and provide detailed insight and analysis on seemingly everything medical. They have locations in New York, London and Beijing, three key geographies to this pandemic.

On March 27, *The Lancet* published an analysis by Dimple D Rajgor, Meng Har Lee, Sophia Archuleta, Natasha Bagdasarian and Swee Chye Quek where they concluded the COVID-19 death rate to be a little worse than the flu but not as bad as the SARS threat a decade earlier:

> *A unique situation has arisen for quite an accurate estimate of the CFR [case fatality rate] of COVID-19. Among individuals onboard the Diamond Princess cruise ship, data on the denominator are fairly robust. The outbreak of COVID-19 led passengers to be quarantined between Jan 20, and Feb 29, 2020. This scenario provided a population living in*

a defined territory without most other confounders, such as imported cases, defaulters of screening, or lack of testing capability. 3711 passengers and crew were onboard, of whom 705 became sick and tested positive for COVID-19 and seven died, 6 giving a CFR of 0·99%. If the passengers onboard were generally of an older age, the CFR in a healthy, younger population could be lower.

Although highly transmissible, the CFR of COVID-19 appears to be lower than that of SARS (9·5%) and Middle East respiratory syndrome (34·4%), but higher than that of influenza (0·1%).[39]

THE GRAND PRINCESS

The Grand Princess launched in 1997. I've been on one cruise, on this ship, and I recall this was the second voyage of the Grand Princess, the largest cruise ship at that time. We took a cruise in the Mediterranean Sea, beginning in Istanbul and ending in Venice. It was a great experience, though cramped in our lower interior room. We had three channels on the little television: a movie channel, a BBC news channel and a channel looping *The Love Boat* episodes, unfortunately the same six episodes for 12 days. The cost of my cruise got bumped with my almost-daily $200 donation to the blackjack table.

The Grand Princess is about the same capacity as the Diamond Princess. On February 11, 2020, the ship sailed out of San Francisco/Oakland to several ports in Mexico. It returned to San Francisco for a next voyage on February 21, bound for Hawaii, Mexico and back to the Bay area. On March 14, 2020, *The Guardian* had a very appropriate headline about this cruise:

From paradise to coronavirus: the Grand Princess and the cruise from hell[40]

A 71-year-old man from California disembarked the February 11 cruise positive with COVID-19 and passed it on to passengers or crew on the February 21 cruise. *The Guardian* reported that the cruise infection was connected to the first positive-tested American from Washington state.[41] About 60 passengers remained on the ship from the February 11 cruise to the February 21 cruise. Back to back cruises on the same ship? Those cruise lovers must have had their fill for a lifetime by the time this unfolded weeks later.

THE CRUISE SHIPS

On March 4, that elderly man from the first cruise died, and the overlap passengers were quarantined by the ship to their rooms. Imagine that experience for a moment: 2,500 passengers able to move about except you; you're not sure what you may have; you're probably getting spotty news reports and you have to contend with all of that confined in a four-hundred-square-foot cabin room.

By now, all passengers knew a bit of what was going on. Again, for the non-quarantined passengers, you don't know how serious it, but it's something big. It's all over the news. You're out of control. You walk around the ship and look at each passenger as if they may be a contagious leper. You see the food you get, and before eating, you're thinking it was prepared by a staff from the previous cruise, sharing rooms, handling your food. You walk up and down stairs, and double take at the handrails. You opt to take an elevator, look at the panel, and put your finger behind your sleeve to touch a button.

You go to your room, stare at the four walls, you turn on the television. The news channel is pounding information on the very crisis you are in. You've exhausted the content on the other channels. You're glued to information but it all feels unsettling. Anxiety is building and while it's not solitary confinement in prison, to a non-prisoner it feels that way.

The ship stayed at sea in the Pacific for four days awaiting its fate by the U.S. government. Anyone stuck in a plane for an hour or two looping around in bad weather waiting to land knows the anxiety. This was for days. Not as confined as an airplane but factoring in the length of time and uncertainty of the virus, a much worse experience.

When the ship entered the San Francisco Bay on March 9, it was covered on the news like the Bronco chase decades earlier. News media painted a picture as if the leper colony from *Ben-Hur* was porting in. But what was actually discovered? Really nothing.

Hundreds were tested, hundreds declined to be tested. Those testing positive or declining tests were sent to be quarantined at various military bases around the country. According to the CDC, 469 people were tested and 16% (78) were positive.[42] Two people, both in their sixties and together, died by the end of the month. Later, a Philippine crew member died in early April.

Two cruise ships offered very controlled environments to observe the spread and impact of the virus. There was medium spread of what we would learn is much more contagious than seasonal flu viruses. It's aggressive to the elderly and those with underlying conditions, primarily respiratory-related, and leaves the younger age groups with flu-like or no symptoms. Later data would show this was much less dangerous to young people than a flu virus.

43

THE AIRCRAFT CARRIERS

Life on an aircraft carrier is in no way similar to the experience of taking a cruise vacation. Sailors live in cramped quarters practicing whatever the opposite of social distancing is. Hallways are cramped and staircases are like going up and down Tee-winot. Most are working long days and not going to the flight deck to enjoy the fresh air breeze and ocean views.

The flight decks are restricted and potentially dangerous so only required and authorized personnel go above deck. Windy conditions and air flow from the jets creates a risky environment requiring much training and structure for the sailors. The flight deck perches 65 feet above the ocean.

In late March, the U.S.S. Theodore Roosevelt ported into Guam and announced a few dozen sailors tested positive for SARS-CoV-2 or COVID-19. Nearly 5,000 people were on board, larger than either of the cruise ship populations. In stark contrast, these were predominantly very healthy, fit young men and women. This provided a very different and still controlled petri dish-type of observation for the spread and impact of COVID-19. Of the group, 840 sailors tested positive for SARS-CoV-2 and 4,098 tested negative. One sailor died from complications associated with COVID-19.[43]

In mid-April 2020, the French announced that their aircraft carrier, Charles de Gaulle, with 2,000 crew members had been infected with the virus. After testing more than 1,700 of the sailors, 940 tested positive for SARS-CoV-2.[44] Thirty-one were hospitalized and one was in intensive care, none died.

Four of the U.S Navy ships ended up with coronavirus outbreaks, with one death and thousands testing positive. This is another sampling of the virus acting like an aggressive flu strain but not as dangerous to the young and healthy. The U.S.S. Theodore Roosevelt data was not critically analyzed for the data demonstrating there was not a significant hospitalization and death threat to the young or those without preexisting conditions.

If you take the data from the cruise ships and aircraft carriers, a broad sampling of ages and health conditions, you have about 14,000 people exposed and 11 fatalities. The rate of infection was much greater than that in the general population. The reason is the tight conditions enabling quick spread. At that rate, of 326,000,000 Americans, we would experience a likely fatality rate of about .07%. That translates to about 228,000 predicative COVID-19 deaths in the United States if the infection rate mirrored the ships, probably not far from where we end up. Those deaths would displace other cause deaths in which case of that, about half may be true all-cause COVID-19 increases. Would America shut down the economy, schools and all societal fabrics if that were the predictive outcome?

CHAPTER 6

THE MODELS

IMPERIAL COLLEGE

The Imperial Institute was created in 1887 in London, as a graduation of the Westminster Hospital Medical School in 1834, the Royal College of Chemistry in 1845, and St. Mary's Hospital Medical School in 1854. Imperial College was officially founded in 1907. *Top Universities* ranked Imperial as the ninth best university in the world with a large emphasis on science and medicine.[45] *U.S. News and World Report* ranked Imperial twentieth worldwide.[46] In 2020, Imperial had a student body of around 20,000, about half in graduate work and half in undergraduate.

Professor Neil Ferguson is the Vice-Dean at the Faculty of Medicine, School of Public Health at Imperial College. Ferguson achieved a master's in physics from Lady Margaret Hall, Oxford and a doctorate in theoretical physics at Linacre College, Oxford. Ferguson has been considered a mathematical and epidemiology expert and authority since his early 30s (born in 1968).

When the swine flu broke out in 2009, he wrote a piece for *The Lancet* called "Closure of schools during an influenza pandemic."[47] In it he opined on school closures as a way to mitigate the spread of the flu and wrote on the opportunity costs on health care workers (for example, figuring out childcare while caring for the sick). Within academic standards, Ferguson was considered a genius at epidemiology and mathematical modeling.

A theory or model embraced by many epidemiologists is called "herd immunity." The idea is that a subset of the population is allowed to or will catch a virus and develop immunity in a tiered way, so not everyone in a community catches it at once and overwhelms the healthcare system. The infected are cared for if necessary, recover, develop antibodies for the virus and then won't spread it or be symptomatic in the future.

Flashback for a moment to 2005. In 2005, there was a breakout of the H5N1 bird flu. Back then, David Nabarro was a senior expert at the World Health Organization. *The Guardian* reported then that Nabarro said the outbreak, which had killed a few dozen people in Asia, could result in a "range of deaths could be anything between five and 150 million."[48] In the same article, Neil Ferguson is quoted with his analysis below.

Quoting *The Guardian*, "Last month Neil Ferguson, a professor of mathematical biology at Imperial College London, told *Guardian Unlimited* that up to 200 million people could be killed. Around 40 million people died in the 1918 Spanish flu outbreak, said Prof Ferguson. There are six times more people on the planet now so you could scale it up to around 200 million people probably."[49] So there's that frame of reference for the Imperial College model author's credibility.

Reaching back a little further, in 2002, there was a potential disease associated with BSE-infected cows and potentially sheep. Professor Ferguson was conducing analysis then and shared this: "Our latest analysis shows that the current risk from sheep could be greater than that from cattle, due to the more intensive controls in place to protect human health from exposure to infected cattle, as compared with sheep. The Imperial College team predicted that the future number of deaths from Creutzfeldt-Jakob disease (vCJD) due to exposure to BSE in beef was likely to lie between 50 and 50,000. In the "worst case" scenario of a growing sheep epidemic, the range of future numbers of death increased to between 110,000 and 150,000."[50] It never happened.

IMPERIAL COLLEGE COVID-19 MODEL

Ferguson authored a COVID-19 model in early March, predicting 500,000 deaths in Great Britain and 2,200,000 deaths in America unless the populace enacted strict social distancing, broad testing and quarantining for those positive with the virus. It became the foundational document and roadmap for Great Britain and the United States, countries that would effectively lock down their citizens to prevent an overwhelming of healthcare facilities all at once.

According to an Imperial College analysis on March 17, they interpreted the model as follows:

In the first scenario, they show that interventions could slow down the spread of the infection but would not completely interrupt its spread. They found this would reduce the demand on the healthcare system while protecting those most at risk of severe disease. Such epidemics are predicted to peak over a three to four-month period during the spring/summer.

In the second scenario, more intensive interventions could interrupt transmission and reduce case numbers to low levels. However, once these interventions are relaxed, case numbers are predicted to rise. This gives rise to lower case numbers, but the risk of a later epidemic in the winter months unless the interventions can be sustained.[51]

As we look at the model in assumptions and its output, here's a quick explanation. Ferguson and his team are among the most expert in this field. It's also easy to pick apart a model that falls apart after the fact. We've all made scaled-to-our-expertise models and assumptions that have failed. We've all had criticism of our work.

Having authored more than a dozen books, I've had some bad reviews and criticisms and it never feels good, especially coming from those who are not experts in the field. I'm quite sure this one will be more of the same. However, this was the most consequential healthcare model ever created. The impacts were both medical in nature and as we would later see, economically impacted billions of people.

The Imperial College report called Report 9: Impact of *non-pharmaceutical interventions* (NPIs) to reduce COVID-19 *mortality and healthcare demand* opens with a callout that the COVID-19 pandemic is the most serious since the Spanish Flu.[52] Options were only suppression and mitigation. Suppression basically says the goal is to limit the reproduction of the virus spread, eliminating person-to-person contact. Mitigation doesn't focus on the spread, but the treatment through drugs, vaccines, etc. as a means to limit the impact.

A do-nothing scenario was predicted by the Imperial College model to result in more than 500,000 COVID-19-related deaths in Great Britain and 2,200,000 deaths in the United States, both peaking in June 2020. Across is their chart, the lower line being the United States.

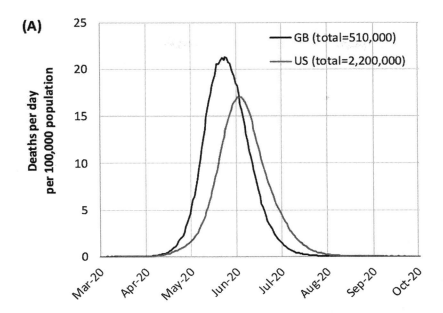

(A)

MODEL ASSUMPTIONS

- *We assumed an incubation period of 5.1 days 9, 10. Infectiousness is assumed to occur from 12 hours prior to the onset of symptoms for those that are symptomatic and from 4.6 days after infection in those that are asymptomatic with an infectiousness profile over time that results in a 6.5-day mean generation time.*

- *On recovery from infection, individuals are assumed to be immune to re-infection in the short term.*

- *Infection was assumed to be seeded in each country [GB and US] at an exponentially growing rate (with a doubling time of 5 days) from early January 2020, with the rate of seeding being calibrated to give local epidemics which reproduced the observed cumulative number of deaths in GB or the US seen by 14th March 2020.*

- *We assume that 30% of those that are hospitalized will require critical care (invasive mechanical ventilation or ECMO) based on early reports from COVID-19 cases in the UK, China and Italy (Professor Nicholas Hart, personal communication).*

- *Based on expert clinical opinion, we assume that 50% of those in critical care will die and an age-dependent proportion of those that do not require critical care die (calculated to match the overall IFR).*

- *We calculate bed demand numbers assuming a total duration of stay in hospital of 8 days if critical care is not required and 16 days (with 10 days in ICU) if critical care is required. With 30% of hospitalized cases requiring critical care, we obtain an overall mean duration of hospitalization of 10.4 days, slightly shorter than the duration from hospital admission to discharge observed for COVID-19 cases internationally13 (who will have remained in hospital longer to ensure negative tests at discharge) but in line with estimates for general pneumonia admissions.*

- *Infection was assumed to be seeded in each country at an exponentially growing rate (with a doubling time of 5 days) from early January 2020, with the rate of seeding being calibrated to give local epidemics which reproduced the observed cumulative number of deaths in GB or the US seen by 14th March 2020.*

- *In the (unlikely) absence of any control measures or spontaneous changes in individual behaviour, we would expect a peak in mortality (daily deaths) to occur after approximately 3 months. In such scenarios, we predict 81% of the GB and US populations would be infected over the course of the epidemic.*

Below are the mathematical projections for hospitalizations and deaths, applied to the United States in a do-nothing scenario:

AGE-GROUP (YEARS)	% SYMPTOMATIC CASES REQUIRING HOSPITALIZATION	% HOSPITALIZED CASES REQUIRING CRITICAL CARE	INFECTION FATALITY RATIO	TOTAL US POPULATION	FATALITIES
0-9	0.1%	5.0%	0.002%	40,000,000	648
10-19	0.3%	5.0%	0.006%	42,000,000	2,041
20-29	1.2%	5.0%	0.03%	45,400,000	11,032
30-39	3.2%	5.0%	0.08%	43,700,000	28,318
40-49	4.9%	6.3%	0.15%	40,600,000	49,329
50-59	10.2%	12.2%	0.6%	42,800,000	208,008
60-69	16.6%	27.40%	2.2%	37,300,000	664,686
70-79	24.3%	43.2%	5.1%	22,700,000	937,737
80+	27.3%	70.9%	9.3%	12,700,000	956,691

Population data from Statista1: https://www.statista.com/statistics/241488/population-of-the-us-by-sex-and-age/

Not all the model assumptions are easily available. One assumption made was that 81% of the population would end up infected. In applying their assumptions to the U.S. population, it predicts a worst-case scenario of 2.8 MM deaths. Imperial College came up with 2.2MM deaths. Uncovering exactly how the 2.2MM number was derived is not broken down in the model released on March 17. The code behind the model was later identified as flawed in a peer group review.[53]

Over the page is their model predicting hospitalizations compared to capacity in the United States. If you look at the "Do nothing" line you can see a peak need for critical care (ICU) hospital beds of approximately 900,000 at one time (~275 x (326,000,000 US population/per 100,000 people)). Even with social distancing, case isolation, quarantining, closing schools, everything, about 300,000 ICU beds would be needed on the peak day.

The lines in descending order are: do nothing; closing schools and universities; case isolation; case isolation and household quarantine; case isolation, home quarantine, social distancing of those over 70, and the bottom flat line is ICU capacity.

U.S. HOSPITAL CAPACITY

According to the American Hospital Association, the United States had the following 2020 hospital capacity:[54]

- **6,146** - total number of all U.S. hospitals
- **924,107** - total staffed beds
- **55,663** - medical-surgical intensive care 4 beds
- **15,160** - cardiac intensive care 5 beds
- **22,721** - neonatal intensive care 6 beds
- **5,115** - pediatric intensive care 7 beds
- **7,419** - other intensive care 9 beds
- **36,353,946** -Total annual admissions in all U.S. hospitals

U.S. hospitals had a total of 924,107 staffed beds and around 90,000 ICU beds in 2020.

Can you see the three-fold ICU shortfall in a best-case scenario and ten-fold shortfall in a do-nothing scenario? This is exactly what led government leaders to panic and not just lockdown businesses and schools, but hospitals and all non-emergency non-COVID-19-related treatment. We later saw this gross miscalculation is

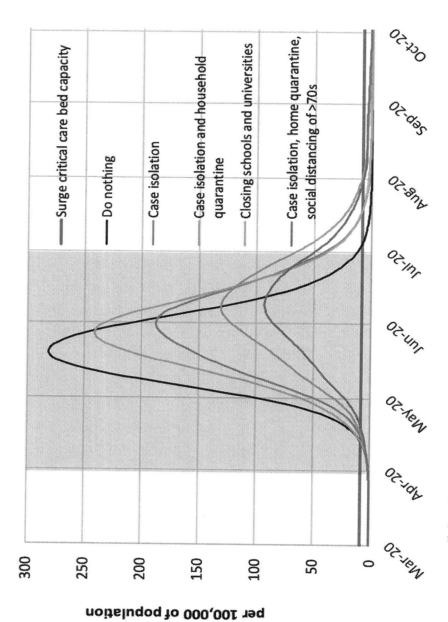

Critical care beds occupied per 100,000 of population

- Surge critical care bed capacity
- Do nothing
- Case isolation
- Case isolation and household quarantine
- Closing schools and universities
- Case isolation, home quarantine, social distancing of >70s

The lines in descending order are: do nothing; closing schools and universities; case isolation; case isolation and household quarantine; case isolation, home quarantine, social distancing of those over 70, and the bottom flat line is ICU capacity.

what triggered the economic collapse as well as a collapse of the healthcare industry.

Hospitals went empty nearly everywhere other than the greater New York City area and a handful in Detroit and New Orleans for about three weeks, creating a vacuum of revenues lost and thousands of healthcare workers laid off, and millions going without their non-COVID-19 treatments.

CRUISE SHIP COMPARISON

However, that model seems implausible given one important actual study we all had access to before this model came out: the cruise ships. The cruise ships provided a perfect analysis of how the virus spreads, who is likely to get infected, hospitalized and who is not likely to survive. Ignoring that data went on to creating the worst world economic collapse in history. Going back to the data from the Diamond Princess cruise ship, this is the demographic spread of the virus:

AGE	PASSENGERS	COVID-19 POSITIVE W/ SYMPTOMS	COVID-19 POSITIVE W/NO SYMPTOMS	DEATHS
0 - 9	16	0	1	0
10-19	23	2	3	0
20 - 29	347	25	3	0
30 - 39	428	27	7	0
40 - 49	334	19	8	0
50 - 59	398	28	31	0
60 - 69	923	76	101	0
70 - 79	1015	95	139	6
80 - 89	216	29	25	1
Totals	3700	301	318	7

The data above is for the Diamond Princess only. Specifics for the Grand Princess are not released at this level of detail, because many did not test. Given the two cruises had nearly identical populations of guests and crew, for this exercise let's extrapolate and double the population spreads of the Diamond Princess to represent both, adding in three deaths from the Grand Princess.

AGE	COMBINED PASSENGERS	ACTUAL CRUISE SHIP DEATHS	IMPERIAL COLLEGE PREDICTIVE DEATHS
0-9	32	0	0
10-19	46	0	0
20-29	694	0	0
30-39	856	0	1
40-49	668	0	1
50-59	796	1	4
60-69	1846	2	33
70-79	2030	6	84
80-89	432	1	33
Totals	**7400**	**10**	**155**

Based on the Imperial College infection rate of .81 and their fatality rate of each age group, the Diamond Princess and Grand Princess cruise ships should have resulted in 155 deaths. Remember, the Imperial College worst-case scenario was in a do-nothing action. This is effectively what happened on the cruise ships because they were infected and spreading before practicing distancing/quarantining and had inferior mitigation capabilities compared to the experience one with symptomatic conditions would receive.

If you consider, and this is a reasonable but hypothetical estimate, that with extra distancing for the elderly and those with pre-existing conditions and better immediate care than those on the cruise ship would get, you get a number of about 5% of the Imperial College estimate, maybe 110,000 potential fatalities compared to 2.2MM. That's a number that is less than a 40% increase from flu deaths in 2017-2018. Would America shut down the entire economy for that prevention, or exercise a strict policy to protect the elderly, care facilities, and those with pre-existing conditions as an address to the virus spread?

According to *The Telegraph*, Professor Ferguson's "report so shook the Prime Minister and his advisers that it reportedly prompted them to shift tack, moving from gradually attempting to achieve "herd immunity" to a lockdown of most businesses, with people only allowed to leave their homes under limited circumstances."[55]

Based perhaps on the Imperial College model, *U.S. News and World Report* reported on March 30, 2020 the following:

"A person's odds for death after infection with the new coronavirus also rose with age. An estimated 0.031% of people in their 20s will die, the new analysis found, compared to 7.8% of people over 80."[56]

- 7.8% of people over 80: 990,000 deaths.
- .031% of people in their 20's: 14,075 deaths.

Someone's laptop needed to be taken away. Or maybe they should take a cruise.

In an ironic closure to Professor Ferguson's role in the pandemic and closures, Ferguson himself would violate the UK lockdown and quarantine order he lectured the public about many times to meet, on more than one occasion, a married woman with whom he was having an affair, resigning in disgrace on May 5, 2020.

On June 2, 2020, Ferguson commented on Sweden's lack of lockdown compared to Great Britain's severe lockdown. His conclusion was that Sweden had the "same effect" as countries that did lockdown, invalidating the effectiveness of the lockdowns.[57]

OXFORD UNIVERSITY

Sunetra Gupta is a professor of Theoretical Epidemiology at Oxford University's Department of Zoology. Gupta graduated from Princeton University in 1987 and later with a doctorate from Imperial College. Shortly after the Imperial College model was released and acted upon, Gupta led an Oxford study refuting the conclusions and predicted the COVID-19 impact would be much less devastating, releasing this just one week after the release of the Imperial College model.

Two core assumptions made the Oxford model much more conservative. First, they assumed only 0.1% of the population was in a high-risk category. Second, they believed that the first transmissions occurred days before the first case was detected. That modeled out to 68% of the population already infected by early March. They also concluded that the epidemics in Italy and the UK began at least a month before the first reported deaths and had already caused a herd immunity situation for most of countries.[58]

What that means is that the UK and, soon to follow, the United States, would enact lockdown measures when the curve was already secured. Reality ended up supporting this model. By the time the United States was locked down, in an effort to slow down the curve, the high point of the deaths was already set in motion and the worst that would come was already in process.

The curve talked about is the steep curve in the models above of ICU capacity that would overwhelm hospitals. This panic is what caused healthcare and political leaders to rush for ventilators and get a Navy ship to New York to cover hospital bed shortfalls. In the end, only New York was overwhelmed, while still not running out of hospital beds and having thousands of ventilators to spare.

As a researcher without medical training, studying this has been a fascinating journey. You will often hear people in the media and in social circles dismiss any-one's opinion if they are not a "subject matter expert." You hear this all the time from the media and from partisan critics. But still, did the model that triggered our economies to shut down and disrupt life of world-history proportions ever make sense? Perhaps being so close to a situation can prevent looking at data and models objectively, looking at conclusions and asking, does this make sense?

The data out of Wuhan was spotty early on, it may be forever in what is widely released. But the data from the cruise ships told us there was no way that there was a materially vulnerable group other than the elderly or those with comorbidities.

Using the word "materially" is a touchy word to use, but it's not fair to 1) play odds for other illnesses and solutions while factoring in a macro-impact, which the medical community and government does all the time, and 2) make the grandest domestic decision in United States history that would crush economies, put tens of millions out of work, prompt domestic violence, stunt student learning, and have countless other impacts.

There is a scene in the movie, *Wargames*, near the end when the missiles were on radar heading for the United States. Barry Corbin's character, General Jack Beringer, was ready to release U.S. missiles on the Soviet Union in response, real missile launches. The man that created the wargames was John Wood's character Dr. Stephen Falken. He leaned into the General and asked if this made any sense and encouraged him to hold off. General Beringer decided it did not make sense and did not launch the missiles. Unfortunately, though it did not make sense for the United States to usher in such severe countermea-sures, those missiles were launched. Incredibly, the overstated model predicting would continue on.

CHANGING THE MODEL

Just hours after Oxford released their model suggesting this would not be the cata-strophic event Imperial predicted, Imperial revised their model down to 20,000 deaths in the UK, with Professor Ferguson qualifying it by stating that half of those victims would probably have died in 2020 of other causes anyway.

On March 25, 2020, a day after Gupta's findings are circulated, Ferguson changed his modeling. Not a tweak, but drastically. *New Scientist* reported on March 25 (March 25!) that Ferguson said *"expected increases in National Health Service capacity and ongoing restrictions to people's movements make him 'reasonably confident' the health service can cope when the predicted peak of the epidemic arrives in two or three weeks. UK deaths from the disease are now unlikely to exceed 20,000, he said, and could be much lower."* [59]

So, in one week's time, one of the most elite and brightest scientists in the world (no sarcasm in that, he was revered as that) changes his forecast from 500,000 deaths to 20,000 or "much lower," a reduction by a factor of 25. It's impossible to accept that social distancing could have such an impact on a model in a week's time.

The timeline for infection to symptoms to hospitalizations to intensive care to death is 10 to 20 or more days. If the model was credible from the beginning, it would take at least two cycles of this to dent it, which means at least a month's time, to see if social distancing was working. The reason is pre-social distancing infections were in motion.

Professors Dr. Eran Bendavid and Dr. Jay Bhattacharya from Stanford University published an article on March 24 in the *Washington Examiner* with a highly skeptical view of the Imperial model and opined that fear was based on bad data rather than probability modeling:

> *"So if 100 million Americans ultimately get the disease, two million to four million could die. We believe that estimate is deeply flawed. The true fatality rate is the portion of those infected who die, not the deaths from identified positive cases."* [60]

More from the *Washington Examiner's* article:

> *The professors cited data from Iceland, China, the United States, and Italy, which is arguably the hardest-hit region when it comes to the coronavirus.*

> *"On March 6, all 3,300 people of Vò were tested, and 90 were positive, a prevalence of 2.7%," the professors said. "Applying that prevalence to the whole province (population 955,000), which had 198 reported cases,*

suggests there were actually 26,000 infections at that time. That's more than 130-fold the number of actual reported cases. Since Italy's case fatality rate of 8% is estimated using the confirmed cases, the real fatality rate could in fact be closer to 0.06%."

"A universal quarantine may not be worth the costs it imposes on the economy, community and individual mental and physical health," the article concluded. "We should undertake immediate steps to evaluate the empirical basis of the current lockdowns."

THE INSTITUTE FOR HEALTH METRICS AND EVALUATION (IHME)

The Institute for Health Metrics and Evaluation (IHME) self-describes as an "independent population health research center at UW Medicine, part of the University of Washington, that provides rigorous and comparable measurement of the world's most important health problems and evaluates the strategies used to address them. IHME makes this information freely available so that policymakers have the evidence they need to make informed decisions about how to allocate resources to best improve population health."

The IHME became an authority of modeling that policy makers used as the United States entered their lockdown (the Imperial College Model prompted the lockdowns) and considered options and likely outcomes.[61] The IMHE model whitepaper detailed their assumptions and predictions on March 30, 2020.[62]

On March 29, 2020, the IHME released a projection of the resources required from that date through the summer of 2020. In it (chart on page 59), they predicted a peak resource need on April 14, 2020. On that summit date, they predicted a need for 232,298 hospital beds, with a shortage of 49,292, and 34,754 ICU beds with an ICU bed shortage of 14,601. Also required would be 18,767 invasive ventilators. Given the capacity listed previously, it's not clear where they saw the huge shortfall.

The IHME model predicted a COVID-19-related death total of anywhere from a low 38,000 to a high 162,000. As an American locked down at the end of March, we're watching the news daily and hearing that just two weeks away we will be crunched with a shortage of hospital capacity and ventilators, an early suspected reason Italy had so many deaths--not enough ventilators.

The closest thing to this model that many Americans are used to is seeing a massive, wide category-five hurricane hurling toward the coast days away, but you

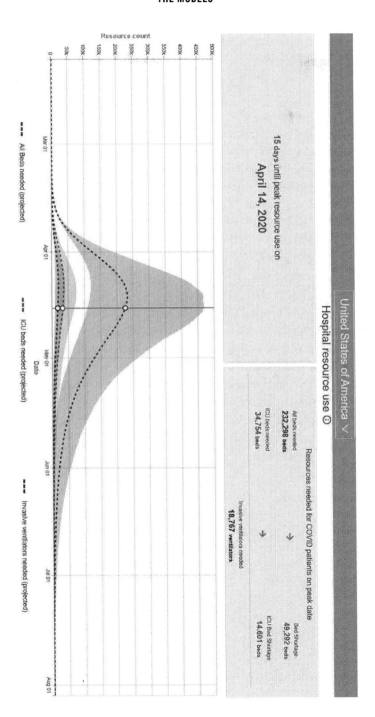

United States of America ∨

Hospital resource use ⓘ

15 days until peak resource use on

April 14, 2020

Resources needed for COVID patients on peak date

All beds needed
232,298 beds

Bed Shortage
49,292 beds

ICU beds needed
34,754 beds

ICU Bed Shortage
14,601 beds

Invasive ventilators needed
18,767 ventilators

Resource count

500k
450k
400k
350k
300k
250k
200k
150k
100k
50k
0

Mar 01   Apr 01   May 01   Jun 01   Jul 01   Aug 01

Date

- - - All Beds needed (projected)

- - - ICU beds needed (projected)

- - - Invasive ventilators needed (projected)

can't leave your beachfront home made of straw. You see it coming and you help-lessly wait with no actions you can take to prevent it. There just isn't enough time.

Except, it would end up a category-one hurricane for the United States (excluding the New York area). On April 1, the model predicted New York state would have 50,000 hospitalizations, while in reality they had 12,226 on April 1, a shortfall by a factor of four.[63] Again, you've got a time lapse between infection and hospitalization and then death. That gap is 10-14 days.

The model was rolled out based on data before the lockdowns occurred. If you lock down on March 20 (New York), the wheels from previous normal social behav-ior would be in motion. Therefore, hospitalizations and death should be close to something predictive and a curve softening would not be realized until the second or later weeks in April. If reality does not deliver, the model inputs are flawed.

The New York Times reported on April 1 that the "number of confirmed or sus-pected coronavirus patients at Cedars-Sinai has grown from about 50 on March 17 to about 115 as of [March 31]."[64] This is a major hospital in Los Angeles with 886 hospital beds. California locked down their state on March 20. Twelve days after the largest state in America, home to 40 million Americans, was locked down, they saw in a major hospital in a major city, an increase of about five hospitalizations per day. Five. Hospitalizations. Per. Day. On top of that, the growth was flat, not exponential like models predicted.

Remember, considering infections occur, a few days pass, then you go to the hospi-tal, that any normal social interactions would be accounted for. Also, remember, cases are not hospitalizations. They are positive tests, where there may be no or only casual symptoms. Non-hospitalized cases are good things, they drive the denominator (deaths/those infected) down and illustrate a lower lethality to the infection.

MODELS IN PLAY

On April 2, 2020, the IHME predicted 56,000 New York state hospitalizations and 11,000 ICU beds while reality was 13,400 hospitalizations and 3,400 ICU beds used. The actual data seen is collapsing to a fraction of the predictions within days, even same day. This was the data used to support extreme economic and social-crushing lockdowns.

April 4, 2020: the IHME predicted for New York state 65,400 hospitalizations and 12,000 ICU beds while reality was 15,905 hospitalizations and 4,100 ICU beds used. The model was consistent to the April 2 model data but shockingly not adjusting for reality. Keep in mind the IHME model from University of Washington created these projections after and accounting for lockdowns, including in New York on March 20.

Imagine following the Major League Baseball (MLB) channel. They are predicting the outcome of a game, but not updating their prediction or presenting the score *during* the game. It would take all of a minute for baseball fans to lose confidence in them, either because they weren't updating the actual score or weren't adjusting outcomes based on what was going on during the game. Perhaps Jonah Hill's character in the movie, *Moneyball*, should join the CDC or IHME. Or some freshman stats student from a local community college.

April 5, 2020: the IMHE model began adjusting data a little more to reality. It reduced the number of peak hospitalizations from 262,000 to 141,000, a 46% reduction in days! ICU needs were reduced at a peak from 39,700 to 29,200, cut by a quarter. Pause for just a moment to consider how large a 46% reduction in hospital capacity needs really is. In a week their prediction was cut almost in half, and this is to where the model was both factoring in lockdown measures and by this date, the course had been set to where lockdowns and social distancing would barely have kicked in yet.

Two days later, the IMHE model revised its data again and new projections were: hospitalizations reduced from 141,000 down to 90,000 and deaths reduced from 80,000 to 60,000. At this point we are now in the territory of fewer COVID-19 deaths than the flu season two years prior. America is now locked down with a depression-level economic ruin as the fallout of state policies.

The important thing to remember about the models is that they factored in all of the preventive measures put in place, including lockdowns and social distancing. The hospitalization models were wrong factoring in these actions, not because they affected and drove down the actuals. Models are just that, but again, common sense from the cruise ship data never supported these models.

I shared a draft of this book with a friend of mine in California. She's progressive and supported the lockdown. After she read this draft, she told me it was eye-opening and she no longer believed the lockdowns were appropriate policy. She did ask me though, was I concerned about being on the right side of history over time. It was an interesting question to ponder.

SARS-CoV-2 was spreading weeks before the lockdowns occurred. The illnesses, hospitalizations and fatalities were in motion before we ever locked down. Had we never locked down, it's highly probable everything that occurred would have anyway. When deaths remained flat to down as states opened up, as people congregated to protest in the memory of George Floyd and nothing happened (cases went up, more on that later), all point to how the models were misused and the lockdowns were the biggest mess in domestic American policy history.

CHAPTER 7

NEW YORK

New York City became the epicenter of the COVID-19 crisis in America. New York City is comprised of five boroughs: Manhattan, Queens, Brooklyn, Staten Island and Bronx. In total New York City has 8.4MM residents and is the most densely populated city in America and one of the most in the world. On average, New York City is home to 27,000 people per square mile, and 765,000 of those residents are over 70 years old, about nine percent.

Manhattan, the center of New York City's five boroughs, is home to 1.4MM of New York City's residents. However, the daytime population in Manhattan is (was) about 4MM people: nearly the 1.4MM residents, more than 1.5MM commuting workers, and the rest visitors or students. People commute into Manhattan daily from as far as Connecticut, New Jersey and Long Island, as well as the other four boroughs. Public transportation is the primary means (80%) to get into the city, with half coming in through the subway, the rest through rail or bus. Around 750,000 people per day route through Grand Central Station, the Beaux-Arts styled landmark opened in 1913, and 24,000 restaurants call Manhattan home, as do 12,000 taxi cabs.

Across the East River is Brooklyn, home to 2.4MM people, the most populated of the five boroughs. Around 35,000 people live there per square mile. Median household income is just under $60,000, and the mean housing unit price is nearly $900,000. With those averages it's not difficult to see that there would be high occupancy per household.

Queens, well known as the home to La Guardia Airport, the New York Mets and the Billie Jean King National Tennis Center (host of the U.S. Open), is also home to 2.3MM people. Median household income is slightly higher than Brooklyn and the average cost of a housing type is $545,000.

The Bronx, home to the New York Yankees, is also home to 1.4MM New Yorkers. Median household income is under $40,000 and their average home price is $400,000. South of Manhattan beyond the Statue of Liberty is Staten Island. Staten Island's 480,000 residents lead the three boroughs outside Manhattan with a median household income of $79,000 and lower home prices, the median at $501,000.

MARCH MILESTONES

March 3, 2020: The first SARS-CoV-2 positive test reached New York on about March 3, 2020.[65]

March 12: Still fewer than 500 COVID-19 cases, Governor Andrew Cuomo rules that gatherings with more than 500 attendees must be cancelled. Broadway theaters shut down.

March 14: The first COVID-19 fatality in New York.

March 16: All schools in New York state closed. At this point, there were about a thousand COVID-19 cases, and seven deaths. All deaths and practically all cases were in the New York City area. Shutting down the rest of the state with no data of any activity outside the New York City metropolitan area was questionable. People with the ability to work from home were ordered to do so.

School closings left 1.25MM kids home and being home-schooled or learning online. It also presented a logistics challenge for hundreds of thousands of parents in the area. In a midwestern suburb of single-family homes it would present a challenge. In the tight quarters of New York, particularly in the Bronx, Queens and Brooklyn, it proved beyond challenging. Many lower income households lacked Wi-Fi, or good Wi-Fi, lacked school supplies, books, and quiet learning-conducive spaces.

Stress would abound in confinement with few getting space to "air out" from each other. Most students need the structure of classroom environments to be disciplined to get through lesson plans. The lockdowns would test students and parents. With the stress of parents not working, or working from home and their kids exercising more needs than usual, the stress placed on families tested everyone.

March 18: New York verified 2,959 positive tests and was ramping up testing,

8,000 tests per day.[66] Neighboring Connecticut, New Jersey and Pennsylvania joined New York in closing shopping malls, parks, bowling alleys, gyms.

March 19: Governor Andrew Cuomo issued an executive order requiring non-essential businesses to reduce staff by 50%. Essential businesses that were exempt from the order include: shipping firms, media, warehousing, grocery and food production, pharmacies, health care providers, utilities, banks and similar financial institutions and companies servicing necessary supply chains.

March 20: Governor Cuomo issued a statewide lockdown order effective March 22. The order shut down non-essential business and personal activity in groups. Shutting down cities like Dallas, Atlanta, Denver, Salt Lake City, is not like shutting down New York. Most cities are suburb-based. Commuters work in either the cities or suburbs and go home to apartments a thousand square feet or more, all the way up to single family homes with a driveway, a yard, green space, and space between residents.

New York City is like a cruise ship: the rooms are small but you're there for life on the decks. Confining New Yorkers to their residences and minimizing outside release was an extreme move that the governor must have considered thoughtfully. This move shows us how serious leaders thought this would be.

HOSPITAL CAPACITY

Approximately 11,000 hospital beds were occupied with COVID-19 patients. New York City has about 20,000 hospital beds. When the analysis was happening in real time, cases and deaths were always reported as the headline grabber. But the real trend indicator of how New York was faring was hospitalizations.

Three crisis issues were identified: hospital beds, ICU beds and ventilators. New York state has a capacity of 53,000 hospital beds, 37,000 ICUs and 3,000 ventilators. A ventilator is a machine that helps people breathe when they can't breathe on their own. A ventilator gets oxygen into the lungs and helps to get rid of carbon dioxide through the lungs. Because a high majority of COVID-19 patients have respiratory issues, you can see the need. ICU-quality ventilators cost from $25,000 to $50,000.[67]

The fear in New York was that they would need ten times the number of current ventilators. In an effort to bridge that gap, the federal government turned to the private sector to help under the Defense Production Act. Back in World War II, Detroit's auto industry halted automobile production and used their plants to produce tanks, aircraft, engines and ammunition. General Motors and its partner Ventec Life Systems, a small maker of ventilators, would be ramped up with a plan of producing thousands by the end of April. As it would turn out, those would not be needed.

Governor Andrew Cuomo made pushes for the 30,000 to 40,000 ventilators needed to handle what he saw as a bulging influx coming. He delivered daily briefings at this point, as were President Trump and his team. President Trump publicly challenged the need for that many ventilators and it sparked controversy in the media.

President Trump said on a television interview on Fox News on April 2, 2020, "I have a feeling that a lot of the numbers that are being said in some areas are just bigger than they're going to be. I don't believe you need 40,000 or 30,000 ventilators."

Cuomo lashed out at the administration that they can "pick up the extra 26,000 people that would die." Those projections were based on a very overstated and flawed IHME model and in the end, New York had many more ventilators than they needed. Noted, Governor Cuomo was cautious and planning for a worst-case scenario based on bad data. The data never really worked when you looked at the most vulnerable only reaching ICU status – the elderly, the obese and those with one or more other pre-existing conditions.

Another fear was a shortage of hospital beds in New York City. Hospitals expanded their capacity but in mid-March, New York leadership felt dire pressure. In reaching out to the federal government, the U.S. Navy hospital ship Comfort arrived to help.

The U.S.N.S. Comfort first launched in 1976. It is a floating hospital of sorts designed to care for combat troops. Nearly three football fields in length, the Comfort serviced troops in the Persian Gulf War, the Iraq War and civilians after Hurricane Katrina's floods ravaged New Orleans. It is supported by more than a thousand crew of medical personnel when active. It sailed into New York on March 30. The initial purpose was to accommodate non-COVID-19 patients as overflow. Fortunately, it wasn't needed and left New York for Virginia in mid-April.

NURSING HOME POLICY – THE ONE DEVASTING MOVE

March 25: The New York Department of Health issued an order to all nursing homes and care facilities requiring them to accept COVID-19 patients to lessen the expected burden on hospitals. It ended up a decision that was reversed in May. This was the single most questionable decision New York made during the pandemic, sending positive-tested patients to comingle with the most vulnerable segment identified. Below is the order:

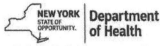

NEW YORK STATE OF OPPORTUNITY.

Department of Health

ANDREW M. CUOMO	HOWARD A. ZUCKER, M.D., J.D.	SALLY DRESLIN, M.S., R.N.
Governor	Commissioner	Executive Deputy Commissioner

DATE: March 25, 2020
TO: Nursing Home Administrators, Directors of Nursing, and Hospital Discharge Planners
FROM: New York State Department of Health

Advisory: Hospital Discharges and Admissions to Nursing Homes

Please distribute immediately to:
Nursing Home Administrators, Directors of Nursing, Directors of Social Work, Hospital Discharge Planners

---

COVID-19 has been detected in multiple communities throughout New York State. There is an urgent need to expand hospital capacity in New York State to be able to meet the demand for patients with COVID-19 requiring acute care. As a result, this directive is being issued to clarify expectations for nursing homes (NHs) receiving residents returning from hospitalization and for NHs accepting new admissions.

Hospital discharge planning staff and NHs should carefully review this guidance with all staff directly involved in resident admission, transfer, and discharges.

During this global health emergency, all NHs must comply with the expedited receipt of residents returning from hospitals to NHs. Residents are deemed appropriate for return to a NH upon a determination by the hospital physician or designee that the resident is medically stable for return.

Hospital discharge planners **must** confirm to the NH, by telephone, that the resident is medically stable for discharge. Comprehensive discharge instructions must be provided by the hospital prior to the transport of a resident to the NH.

No resident shall be denied re-admission or admission to the NH solely based on a confirmed or suspected diagnosis of COVID-19. NHs are prohibited from requiring a hospitalized resident who is determined medically stable to be tested for COVID-19 prior to admission or readmission.

Information for healthcare providers on COVID-19 is readily available on the New York State Department of Health public website at https://coronavirus.health.ny.gov/information-healthcare-providers. As always, standard precautions must be maintained, and environmental cleaning made a priority, during this public health emergency.

Critical personal protective equipment (PPE) needs should be immediately communicated to your local Office of Emergency Management, with the appropriate information provided at the time of request. Requests **MUST** include:

   o Type and quantity of PPE by size;
   o Point of contact at the requesting facility or system;
   o Delivery location;
   o Date request is needed to be filled by; AND
   o Record of pending orders.

Thank you for your ongoing support and cooperation in responding to COVID-19. General questions or comments about this advisory can be sent to covidnursinghomeinfo@health.ny.gov.

Empire State Plaza, Corning Tower, Albany, NY 12237 | health.ny.gov

As we look to Dr. Fauci and the CDC for guidance on what we should do in balancing locking down, reopening, and the social and economic consequences, a question comes to mind: Where the hell were the "experts" when states (it wasn't just New York, it was many) decided to require nursing homes take COVID-19 patients and that all care workers in those facilities were not required to be tested? It's easy for Governor Cuomo's critics to blame him, but doesn't the blame reside with the health "experts" that should have seen this coming? This is why we should all look at data ourselves and not simply follow the media like sheep.

CONTINGENCY PLANS

March 27: Another overflow facility created was the Javits Center. The Javits Center opened in 1986 alongside the Hudson River. With 760,000 square feet of floor space and hosting 40,000 companies a year for events, it's the largest convention center in the country. It may be best known for hosting the Hillary Clinton 2016 campaign event the night of the presidential election. It was converted into a makeshift hospital to care for overflow COVID-19 patients. The facility was set up to accommodate 1,000 patients, four groups of 250 into 40,000 square feet areas each. Capacity grew to 1,700 and never saw more than 50 COVID-19 patients.

Nadia, a four-year-old tiger at the Bronx Zoo, tested positive for COVID-19 after exhibiting a cough. It's believed she caught it from a zoo employee.

March 28: New York City reached a single day peak of 1,629 new hospitalizations. The daily hospitalizations are a cumulative effect though. Each day eats up capacity because an average stay was up to seven days to survive and get released, or not survive. It's a fascinating and scary observation, this pandemic, how it sweeps through quickly, infects a plurality of the population and then disappears.

President Trump was criticized mightily for stating on February 28 that the virus and illnesses would just "disappear like a miracle," accused of being tone deaf. But by late spring we saw just that. Georgia saw this two weeks after they reopened. It's very similar to imagining a tornado sweeping through, wreaking havoc and then it's gone. Most deaths that occurred after April were relegated to those in nursing home or long-term care facilities. COVID-19 would be dangerous throughout 2020 but not like the wave that hit New York in March and April.

APRIL MOVES

April 1: Playgrounds closed to address lack of compliance to social distancing mandates.

April 6: Fines for violating social distancing guidelines increased to a maximum $1,000. At this date, New York was at its peak cases, hospitalizations and fatalities. Within two weeks, the crisis was all but over. Not cases, hospitalizations and fatalities, but those combined as a crisis.

April 7: Fatalities are always a lagging indicator of progress. Fatalities peaked at 538 (real-time fatalities, not backdated ones). Within a week that daily number halved and a week after that down to almost zero.[68] Cumulatively, New York had lost 5,500 people.

April 18: By the time the wave was past New York City, Mayor Bill de Blasio threw a little gas on the stress-fire people were feeling. On April 18, the mayor would tweet out on Twitter a suggestion for those not practicing social distancing. In the video he posted, he said:

> *"Thank you to everyone who has done this the right way, but we still know there's some people who need to get the message," de Blasio said. "And that means sometimes making sure the enforcement is there to educate people and make clear we've got to have social distancing. So, now it is easier than ever — when you see a crowd, when you see a line that's not distanced, when you see a supermarket that's too crowded, anything, you can report it right away so we can get help there to fix the problem."*

De Blasio encouraged New Yorkers to report and send pictures of those not practicing social distancing, shaming their neighbors. Knowing that New York was well through the worst of it, it seemed pointless to encourage neighbors to turn on each other. That said, as we will see later, de Blasio critics have been quoted as saying the mayor "has blood on his hands" for his handling of the COVID-19 outbreak, an absurd accusation.

One justification was de Blasio's reluctance early on to close schools. Data supported that children and young people are at virtually no risk of COVID-19 and have a very low ability to pass the virus on to others. There is no action de Blasio could have taken to materially affect the course New York was on.

Resources never ended up depleted and New Yorkers simply had to get through the deck fate dealt them.

April 20: New York lost 96 people and a total of 9,944 from the pandemic-to-date. Deaths are sharply declined, as did cases and hospitalizations. At this point it is just a matter of time to get back to a new normal. Four weeks into the lockdown, with cases, hospitalizations and fatalities subsiding, and warmer weather arriving in New York, getting outdoors would give these families and students some reprieve and much needed space out of their homes.

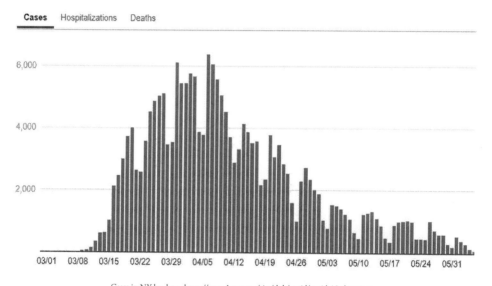

Cases in NY by date: https://www1.nyc.gov/site/doh/covid/covid-19-data.page

NEW YORK

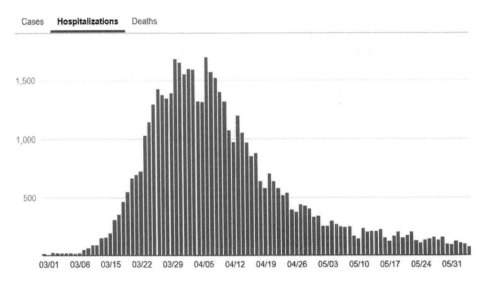

New Hospitalizations in NY by date: https://www1.nyc.gov/site/doh/covid/covid-19-data.page

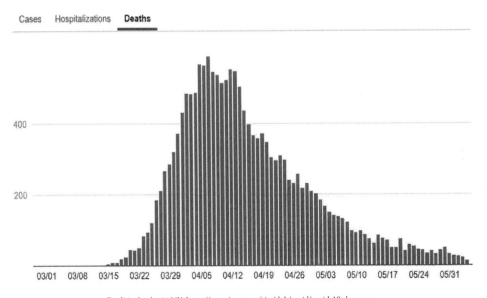

Fatalities by day in NY: https://www1.nyc.gov/site/doh/covid/covid-19-data.page

NEW YORK COVID-19 DEMOGRAPHICS

Within the most affected neighborhoods in Brooklyn, Queens and the Bronx, about 20% of the residents live in dwellings that house two or more people per room. Around 60% of the areas with the most COVID-19 cases overlap with a high number of residents per space. COVID-19, based on case results through both the United States and Europe, predominately spreads within the family or within a hospital or care facility. It's spread by close contact; there aren't SARS-CoV-2 viruses flying through the outdoor air like spring pollen.

If you consider those three elements, you can see why New York was hit harder than other cities. High density dwellings and living spread SARS-CoV-2 more than less dense communities, and then with infected people congesting few hospitals, a domino of spreading followed.

Minorities were disproportionately affected by COVID-19. Black and Hispanic residents make up half of the city's population but made up more than 60% of the fatalities. It's not a huge disparity, but it is accurate that comorbidity exists more within minorities, with conditions such as hypertension and diabetes.

Cases were most concentrated in the outer areas of Brooklyn, Queens and Bronx. One note though: cases are not the measuring stick. It's likely as more testing is done that up to half of all New York City residents may end up positive, maybe more. Most positive cases are asymptomatic or lightly symptomatic. The CDC stated in June that asymptomatic people are highly unlikely to transmit. Measuring hospitalizations from these geographies is most insightful. Higher income Manhattan recorded many fewer cases than the outer boroughs. Curiously, Harlem experienced fewer cases than outer boroughs and is densely populated.

FATALITY DEMOGRAPHICS

New York ended up with the following age distribution of COVID-19 fatalities:

- 80 and older (38%)
- 70-79 (27%)
- 60-69 (20%)
- 50-59 (10%)

- 40-49 (3.7%)
- 39 and younger (2%)[69]

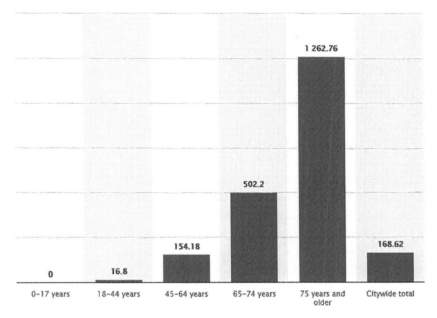

Source: https://www1.nyc.gov/site/doh/covid/covid-19-data.page

NEW COVID-19 PATIENTS CONTRACTING THE VIRUS AT HOME	
Underlying health condition	96%
51 or older	73%
Contracted at home	66%
Unemployed	46%
African American/Latino	45%
Retired	37%

Source: State of New York data and The New York Times

Nearly all COVID-19 deaths occurred in those with preexisting medical conditions that made them more vulnerable to the disease, including diabetes, asthma, lung disease, cancer and immunodeficiency. A whopping 96% of hospitalizations and deaths were to those with underlying conditions: 93% were over 65, 66% over 75, and virtually none under those ages died without preexisting conditions.

WHY NEW YORK?

New York ended up with a much higher percentage of SARS-CoV-2 cases and COVID-19 fatalities in the United States than its share of the population. Why they experienced the blow-up that no other city did is a question everyone asked throughout the spring and summer of 2020. While no one will ever know for certain, the most compelling reasons are:

- Travel hub for domestic and international travel, so the spread was likely from more sources at the same time
- Large family sizes living in close quarters
- Heavy reliance on public transportation
- Government policy requiring positive cases be sent to nursing homes and long-term care facilities

Of the cases New York received, who was most vulnerable? Christopher Petrilli of the NYU Grossman School led a team of colleagues on just this analysis. Their paper is titled *"Factors associated with hospitalization and critical illness among 4,103 patients with COVID-19 disease in New York City,"* published on April 11, 2020.[70] In it they uncovered:

- *Among 4,103 Covid-19 patients, 1,999 (48.7%) were hospitalized, half of whom were discharged home, and 292/1,999 (14.6%) died or were discharged to hospice*
- *Of 445 patients requiring mechanical ventilation, 162/445 (36.4%) have died*
- *Strongest hospitalization risks were age ≥75 years, age 65-74, and heart failure*
- *In the decision tree for admission, the most important features were age >65 and obesity*
- *Conclusions: Age and comorbidities are powerful predictors of hospitalization; however, admission oxygen impairment and markers of inflammation are most strongly associated with critical illness*

The pronounced takeaway that is unique to other studies released to this date is the impact obesity has on a patient's likelihood of a hospitalization or more. In thinking of why Japan (no lockdown) had such a low fatality rate per population, it looks important to factor in low obesity in the far east.

Of 191 countries ranked, below are some of the rankings and the percent of obese within the population:

- 189 – India, ranked near the bottom (best) with 3.9% of their population obese. Between this and their low elderly population you can 1) see why their COVID-19 fatalities and even cases were so low, as well as fatalities and 2) question why this poor country locked down so heavily.
- 185 – Japan at 4.3%
- 106 – Italy at 19.9%
- 96 – Sweden at 20.6%
- 12 – United States at 34.6%[71]

Though not on this list, South Korea has an obesity rate about equal to Japan, a contributing reason South Korea fared well throughout the COVID-19 pandemic.

LOCKDOWN FALLOUT

POLITICS

The two leaders at the front of the epicenter in New York were Mayor Bill de Blasio and Governor Andrew Cuomo. Both played key roles in managing the crisis and each ended up with very different public perceptions of their handling of the New York crisis.

In the fourth quarter of 2019, *Morning Consult* published an approval rating for each governor, other than those just elected in November 2019.[72]

The top ten rated governors by approval rating were Republicans:

1. Mark Gordon (R - WY) 69%
2. Larry Hogan (R - MD) 69%
3. Charlie Baker (R - MA) 69%
4. Phil Scott (R - VT) 65%
5. Chris Sununu (R - NH) 59%
6. Doug Burgum (R - ND) 58%
7. Ron DeSantis (R - FL) 58%
8. Greg Abbott (R - TX) 58%

9. Asa Hutchinson (R - AR) 58%
10. Kay Ivey (R - AL) 58%

Other noted Governors:
- Gretchen Whitmer (D-MI) 42%
- Gavin Newsom (D-CA) 42%
- Andrew Cuomo (D-NY) 47%
- Kate Brown (D-OR) 37%

After running for the Democrat nomination for president in 2019, and withdrawing in September, Mayor Bill de Blasio had an approval rating of 33%.[73] By public accounts, early on Mayor deBlasio saw the COVID-19 pandemic more casually than others. As hospitals saw an increase year over year of flu-like cases (1,156 in 2020 compared to 422 in 2019) on March 12, de Blasio was communicating and desiring that New Yorkers continue on with business as usual and leaving schools open.[74]

De Blasio and Cuomo were at odds on degrees of lockdowns early on for New Yorkers. De Blasio, a liberal progressive, shared concerns over schooling, lunches they provide for poorer families, and employment for his city. The day after schools closed, he caught some media fire for going to the gym and not practicing social distancing.

Cuomo became a face of the COVID-19 crisis and his approval rating and national reputation soared in March and April. Delivering lengthy daily morning briefings broadcast nationally, he talked tough, matter-of-fact, demonstrated empathy and spoke with a tightness de Blasio lacked. Cuomo became governor in 2010, and prior to that was a prosecutor, New York state attorney general and federal housing secretary. He entered this crisis in his third term as governor.

In an April Siena College Research Institute poll, 87% of New Yorkers approved of how Cuomo was handling the crisis.[75] In a Democrat-dominated state, it's not surprising he would far exceed President Trump's approval rating in the same poll by more than 40 percentage points. This was his highest approval rating in seven years in office. A crisis can do that, where President George W. Bush achieved his highest approval ratings in the year following the 9/11 attacks.

With the 2020 presidential election looming months away, the Democrat party was divided on Joe Biden's competency and probability of getting elected. The party was divided between far-left progressives desiring more socialist-like policies championed by Senator Bernie Sanders, and former vice president Joe Biden, who was often incoherent in his interviews. With party members weighing alternatives for the now-delayed democrat convention to August, Cuomo's presidential-like appearance sparked momentum that he may end up the democrat nominee.

Below are some headlines capturing the moment:

"What the 'Cuomo 2020' fantasy says about 2020 reality"[76]

"Unloved by progressives, New York's Andrew Cuomo has the spotlight now"[77]

"'President Cuomo' is new daydream for those fretting over Biden"[78]

"Andrew Cuomo for president? Joe Biden could make it happen"[79]

"Andrew Cuomo supporters quietly angling him for 2020 vice president gig"[80]

"Cuomo supporters reportedly pushing NY governor as Biden running mate"[81]

"Draft Cuomo 2020 groundswell emerges amid the New York governor's coronavirus response"[82]

Governor Cuomo shut down rumors and talk of running for national office in 2020. It's interesting how the crisis thrust Cuomo into the national spotlight and elevated his status.

THE REST OF NEW YORK

While New York City struggled, the rest of the state was in limbo. There were no significant cases, hospitalizations or fatalities due to COVID-19. Cuomo stated in March that it was too difficult to have a stay-in-place policy for the greater New York City area and not for the rest of the state. Still, the data was not supporting any crisis anywhere in New York outside the New York City metropolitan area.

Onondaga County includes the entire Syracuse area. Onondaga County barely felt a bump in healthcare activity. Onondaga had fewer than 700 positive cases (a fraction of which were hospitalized; their peak was under 50) and 22 deaths through April 23, when New York City was well over their peak. Meanwhile, hospitals were empty. With only emergencies and COVID-19 illnesses serviced in practically all hospitals nationwide, hospitals and local healthcare providers were going broke.

In Erie County, home to Buffalo, New York, similar reality. With a population of nearly a million people, they had a cumulative 2,300 positive cases through late April 2020 and 164 deaths. While the death-to-case ratio looks high, it's likely with more tests the ratio was much lower, similar to what we later saw in most communities as testing became broader.

New Yorkers started to unwind at the end of April. People were seen in Central Park, walking the streets, walking through Times Square. If any city in the world needed a reprieve, it was New York. Hospitalizations dropped off, COVID-19 deaths, real-time deaths, not backdated ones, dropped dramatically. It was time to breathe again.

On April 28, a group of Jewish people would congregate for a funeral. Mayor Bill de Blasio got wind of this and send this tweet out on Twitter:

> *My message to the Jewish community, and all communities, is this simple: the time for warnings has passed. I have instructed the NYPD to proceed immediately to summons or even arrest those who gather in large groups. This is about stopping this disease and saving lives. Period.*[83]

New York still had a way to go to get back to normal.

CHAPTER 8

AROUND THE WORLD IN 30 DAYS

At the time New York and America were locking down, much of the world was a week or two ahead and in full swing of COVID-19 hospitalizations and suppression methods.

EUROPE

Beginning with Europe below are the lockdown measures governments exercised to "flatten the curve" of infections and ultimately hospitalizations. Flattening the curve means, if you go back to the models, avoiding the big peak of hospitalizations that overwhelm resources.

   While reviewing lockdown measures various countries took, and the cases and COVID-19 deaths recorded, it may be helpful for you to glance back at respective populations for context and scale.

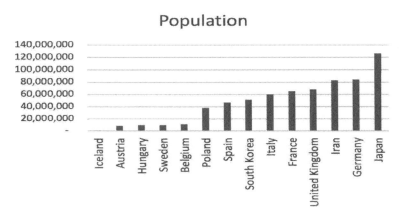

Below is a chart illustrating COVID-19 fatalities-per-million, an important context because absolute fatalities without a balance of overall populations is meaningless to compare.

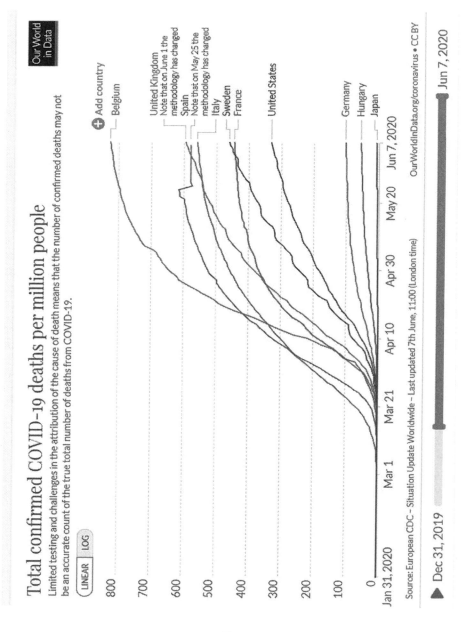

Total confirmed COVID-19 deaths per million people

Limited testing and challenges in the attribution of the cause of death means that the number of confirmed deaths may not be an accurate count of the true total number of deaths from COVID-19.

Source: European CDC – Situation Update Worldwide – Last updated 7th June, 11:00 (London time)   OurWorldInData.org/coronavirus • CC BY

ITALY

Italy realized one of the most challenging COVID-19 illness and fatality experiences in the world. They had one of the first and rapid breakouts in their northern country. Italy locked down the entire country on March 9. Non-essential businesses and schools were closed. Like in America, grocery stores, gas stations and pharmacies remained open.

Travel within the country was banned unless necessary. If Italian residents sought to leave their homes, they had to print out certificates with the reason so that could be shared with the police if stopped. It's not quite martial law, but the closest we'd seen since World War II.

Italy has a fairly older-skewed population, particularly in the north. Nearly a quarter of their population is over 65. As we saw earlier, Italy lost on average the last few years 17,000 lives to the flu. If you consider likely overlap between influenza and COVID-19 infection during March and April 2020, they ended up in a predicable place.

There was news that due to resource constraints Italy was also prioritizing caring for the young over the elderly. This headline ran in *Business Insider* in March: *Faced with tough choices,* "Italy is prioritizing young COVID-19 patients over the elderly."

ITALY'S HEALTHCARE SYSTEM
Below is a comparison of Italy's healthcare system compared to the United States, offered by Nationmaster.

STATISTIC	ITALY	UNITED STATES
Accuracy and completeness in filling out reports	66.76; ranked 25th	74.35; ranked 11th, 11% more than Italy
Convenient location	70.28, ranked 33rd	80.1, ranked 12th, 14% more than Italy
Cost	68.02, ranked 20th , 48% more than United States	45.81, ranked 41st
Friendliness and courtesy of staff	58.06, ranked 31st	74.92, ranked 11th, 29% more than Italy

Health care system index	64.54, ranked 27th	69.03, ranked 23rd, 7% more than Italy
Modern equipment	88.6, ranked 24th	95.58, ranked 11th, 8% more than Italy
Short waiting times	39.44, ranked 37th	60.5, ranked 10th, 53% more than Italy
Skill and competence of medical staff	70, ranked 23rd	74.69, ranked 16th, 7% more than Italy
Speed in delivering examinations and reports	51.67, ranked 34th	69.57, ranked 14th, 35% more than Italy

Every category is ranked below the United States. The structure is quite different from that in America. Healthcare in Italy is funded through (mostly) payroll taxes. It's then no charge to visit a doctor for standard visits, but for lab work and prescriptions there are copays. Elderly are exempt from any charges.

As exhibited in the chart above, it can be a much longer wait time to see a doctor or receive care; getting an appointment can take months. Imagine how that would go over in America. Also, with congested options in southern Italy, many southern residents flock up north for quicker service.

COVID-19 CARE

A quote from an article in *The Independent* on March 13:

> *"A doctor in Italy has told The Independent how medics there are being forced to ration care to patients in the wake of the coronavirus outbreak with elderly patients being denied care based on their age and whether they have other conditions. Official guidance to doctors in Italy, seen by The Independent, have said only patients 'deemed worthy of intensive care' should get it and decisions based on a 'distributive justice' approach balancing the demand for care versus available resources. I know from talking to colleagues in Lombardia, the most affected region in Italy, that they are using a cut off of 65-years-old in case of pre-existing comorbidities. In Bologna, we are working with 80-years-old as our cut off, but between 65 and 80-years-old we still consider comorbidities." [84]*

The Italian College of Anesthesia, Analgesia, Resuscitation and Intensive Care (SIAARTI) established criteria for a hierarchy of how patients would be treated. Treatment for the elderly and others with health conditions factored in the patient's likelihood of survival and life expectancy.

Would ubiquitous care for the elderly and those with comorbidities have reduced their fatalities? Only those in the scene would know but it sure appears that way.

Below are two charts illustrating COVID-19 cases and deaths at the time Italy began to relax their lock down and get back to normal.

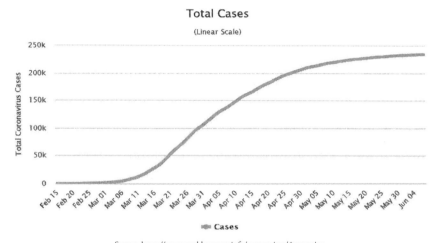

Source: https://www.worldometers.info/coronavirus/#countries

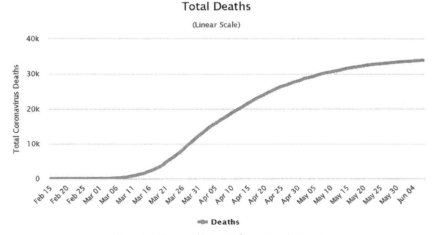

Source: https://www.worldometers.info/coronavirus/#countries

Below is the age distribution of COVID-19 deaths in Italy:

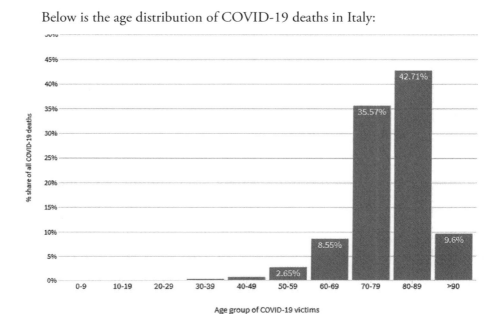

Source: https://www.statista.com/statistics/1105061/coronavirus-deaths-by-region-in-italy/

Italy realized one of the highest per capita COVID-19 deaths of all western countries (if you factor in counting methods). The median age of fatalities was 82. Italy acted late on addressing vulnerabilities in nursing homes. The first case was identified on January 21, and their first guideline for nursing homes was issued on March 9, well into the spread. Nursing homes were not prioritized with personal protective equipment, nor was testing for staff.

Attention was focused on acute care centers, hospitals, not on elderly facilities. Like we saw in America, it was the one controllable element that went unnoticed by nearly all leaders at the time of the lockdowns. About half of those people who lost their lives were infected in or through nursing homes and long-term care facilities. Italy began reopening their society and businesses on May 5, 2020.

UNITED KINGDOM

Britain locked down on March 23, implementing a model closer to Germany than Italy or Spain. Commuting to work, travel to essential businesses and solitary exercise outside was permitted and not restricted by time (France) or requiring papers (Spain and Italy).

Healthcare in the United Kingdom is called the National Health Service (NHS). In short, everyone has the same healthcare and it's a government service. It's comparable to the "Medicare For All" talk in America. A downside is that many treatments are not available "in network" that could save lives or extend the life of a patient. It's a cost-benefit decision. Generally speaking, the NHS covers healthcare for immigrants too, whether refugees, asylum seekers, etc. The two charts below illustrate COVID-19 cases and deaths at the time the UK began to relax their lock down and get back to normal.

Total Cases
(Linear Scale)

Source: https://www.worldometers.info/coronavirus/#countries

Total Deaths
(Linear Scale)

Source: https://www.worldometers.info/coronavirus/#countries

The UK suffered one of the highest per capita COVID-19 deaths in the west. Like Italy, the median age of fatalities was 82, and three-fourths were over 75. An estimated 8,000 of their 32,000 COVID-19 deaths by mid-May, one quarter, were in nursing homes. England began reopening in late May.[85]

FRANCE

While France initially thought their first COVID-19 case was in 2020, evidence in May proved that the first known case of COVID-19 was in December 2019, likely in the third week. The victim had not traveled so it's unclear how he contracted it. France locked down the entire country on March 17, mirroring the Italian orders including citizens documenting why they left home.

French residents had to document when they would come and go and were limited to one hour outside the home. It was luxurious solitary confinement: staying in your place twenty-three hours a day and one hour outdoors. Fines were exercised for those who broke these rules.

France was one of the harder hit EU countries in fatalities per capita. Around 94% of COVID-19 fatalities were 65 or older. Schools began reopening on May 12, as well as other businesses. Below are the COVID-19 case and death totals at the time they began reopening:

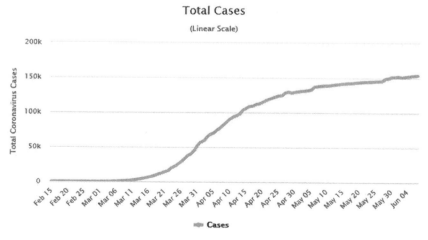

Total Cases
(Linear Scale)

Source: https://www.worldometers.info/coronavirus/#countries

Total Deaths

(Linear Scale)

Source: https://www.worldometers.info/coronavirus/#countries

BELGIUM

Belgium began their lockdown on March 18. Belgium, home to the European Union headquarters, implemented a lockdown similar to France except without the papers. Belgium was hit with the highest per capita fatality rate within the entire EU. Why? Data integrity. Unlike other countries early on, Belgium was counting all potential COVID-19 deaths in nursing homes, even if they did not test positive for SARS-CoV-2.

Politico reported that of Belgium's "official" COVID-19 deaths, "44 percent died in hospital (and were tested). The majority 54 percent died in a nursing home — and only in 7.8 percent of those cases was COVID-19-confirmed as the cause." We will discuss data integrity later. It's very curious why Belgium chose a different inclusion method than other EU countries. At this point, to get an accurate number, you almost have to ballpark based on all-cause mortality averages year over year.

The case and death totals for Belgium well after they began reopening businesses on May 11 and schools on May 18 are on the opposite page.

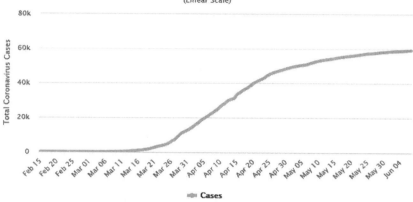

Total Cases

(Linear Scale)

Source: https://www.worldometers.info/coronavirus/#countries

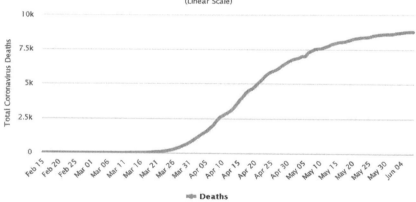

Total Deaths

(Linear Scale)

Source: https://www.worldometers.info/coronavirus/#countries

GERMANY

Germany did not lock down their residents. On March 22, they rolled out strict social distancing rules. Many non-essential businesses were ordered to shut down. Gatherings of more than two were banned except for families. Some German states (Bavaria and Saarland) exercised stricter lockdown measures than others. Commuting to work was still permitted. Businesses that enable patrons to be 1.5 meters apart were permitted to remain open.

Germany began reopening on May 1. Below are the case and death totals for Germany at the time they began reopening.

SPAIN

Spain locked down the entire country on March 14. They materially followed the ban Italy did, and their military and police enforced it in a way not seen in America. Understanding Belgium's unvalidated counting of COVID-19 fatalities and that the UK changed their counting, Spain had the highest per capita death rate within the EU, perhaps highest anywhere.

Around 95% of COVID-19 fatalities were in people 70 and older. And 80% of the population lives in urban areas, which could account for faster spread and a stress on healthcare capacity, like New York experienced.

Spain began reopening on May 2nd in a four-tier approach with the plan of fully reopening by mid-June. Below are the case and death totals for Spain well after they began reopening.

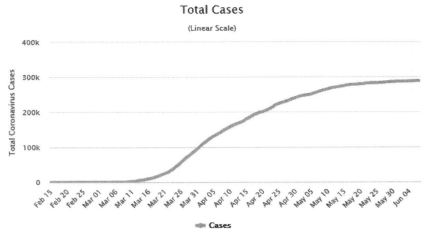

Source: https://www.worldometers.info/coronavirus/#countries

Total Deaths

(Linear Scale)

Source: https://www.worldometers.info/coronavirus/#countries

SWEDEN

By far the most interesting case study of all, Sweden declined to lock down. Fortunately, we have a control group case study with which to compare their "curve" and death rate compared to peer European countries. Gatherings of more than 50 people were banned on March 29. No one was to visit a nursing home after March 31. Still, schools, gyms, bars and restaurants stayed open throughout the spread of the pandemic. Instead, the government urged citizens to act responsibly and follow social distancing guidelines.

From a social distancing perspective, more than half of Swedes live alone, unique, with a very large work-from-home workforce. With a much mellower approach to navigating the SARS-CoV-2 outbreak, there is little doubt that Sweden will face lighter economic consequences than other countries. Germany too. In fact, their economy expanded slightly in the second quarter of 2020. Consider the recovery for Spain and Italy, both with struggling economies before the outbreak and now contending with a complete military-like shutdown.

Swedish leadership had the foresight to do what few countries were bold enough to do. They balanced risk and consequence, figured that the spread would happen and would not overwhelm their healthcare capacity. Suppression tactics like lockdowns would not change the outcome, and the consequence of locking down their economy would do more balanced harm than good. The United States did not have that luxury.

The case and death totals for Sweden in early June as fatalities were leveling off are on the next page.

AROUND THE WORLD IN 30 DAYS

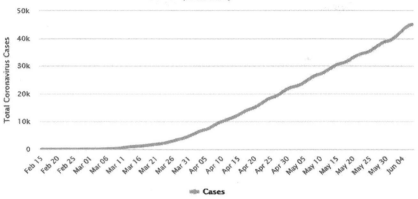

Total Cases
(Linear Scale)

Source: https://www.worldometers.info/coronavirus/#countries

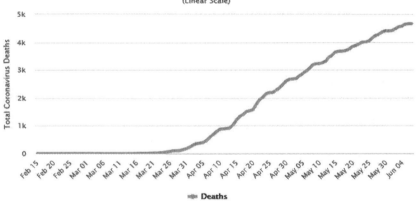

Total Deaths
(Linear Scale)

Source: https://www.worldometers.info/coronavirus/#countries

Below is the age distribution of COVID-19 deaths in early May 2020:

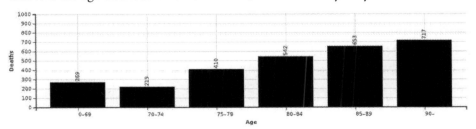

The median age of Sweden's fatalities was 83. Sweden's model (and Japan's) would be the center of worldwide controversy. Most would criticize Sweden, and those opposing strict lockdowns, or supported early reopening's, would tout Sweden as the standard from which to measure. The critics would say that neighboring Finland (50 deaths per million) and Norway (41 deaths per million) far outperformed Sweden (328 deaths per million).

On May 30, Norway's Prime Minister Erna Solberg reflected back on the lockdowns and said this: "Was it necessary to close schools? Perhaps not." [86] She embraced the Swedish model.

Proponents said Sweden was in the same general average as most western European countries, the median age of their victims was 83 and nearly all had preexisting conditions, were above life expectancy and many living in care facilities. With that average result to western Europe, they maintained their economy and schooling. There is no right or wrong answer, it's a risk and consequence balance and opinion. You be the judge.

HUNGARY

Hungary closed its borders on March 17. On March 26, they implemented a lockdown barring indoor and outdoor gatherings, but other than maintaining social distancing, Hungarians were able to go to work, shop and go outdoors. It is an interesting case study to follow since they exercised lighter lockdown measures than most of their EU peers.

Hungary had 425 COVID-19 deaths by the time they began reopening on April 29, 44 deaths per million and among the lowest in the world. The case and death totals for Hungary in early June are on the next page.

Total Cases

(Linear Scale)

Source: https://www.worldometers.info/coronavirus/#countries

Total Deaths

(Linear Scale)

Source: https://www.worldometers.info/coronavirus/#countries

JAPAN

Japan's first COVID-19 death was on February 12. Like Sweden, Japan opted not to undergo a lockdown. Japan has a population density of 900 people per square mile. For comparison, the United States has 93, Italy has 533, California has 253, Florida has 400 and New York City has 27,000.

Prime Minister Shinzo Abe gave closure options to governors and shop owners. Unlike most other countries, restaurants, businesses, factories, hotels and public transportation remained open. Schools closed, a little ironic since data showed children, if not immune, were certainly not vulnerable to SARS-CoV-2. Critics argued the Japanese leadership put the economy in higher precedence than health care.

If you read articles from that time, you will see critics cite an increasing number of cases, which is an illogical argument. By early April, anyone following the pandemic ascertained there was a multiple of ten to a hundred actual cases versus what was reported, and that validating cases was a good thing, demonstrating a higher denominator and therefore very low fatality rate.

Cases don't matter as much as the trend in hospitalizations and ICUs required. Japan realized one of the lowest per capita fatality rates (7 per million people), the number that really matters, the ultimate scorecard for evaluating how countries fared compared to one another.

Below are the case and death totals for Japan in early June.

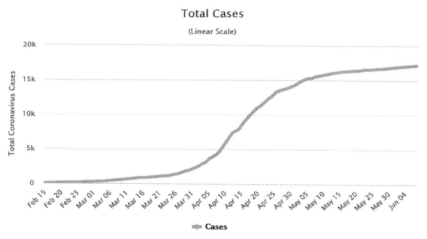

Source: https://www.worldometers.info/coronavirus/#countries

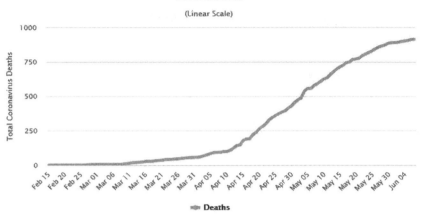

Total Deaths

(Linear Scale)

Source: https://www.worldometers.info/coronavirus/#countries

SOUTH KOREA

South Korea was widely hailed in the media as a model country in their handling of SARS-CoV-2. They were very aggressive testing for the virus out of the gate. Within a week of their first positive test on their homeland, the South Korean government worked closely with the private healthcare industry to create mass testing. A week-plus later, thousands of test kits were shipped daily.

South Korea also quickly identified a city called Daegu, a city about the size of Austin, TX, as a source of spread. South Korea did not lock down but rather exercised an intensive social distancing campaign to mitigate the quick spread. South Korea never experienced a Lombardy (Italy)-like outbreak and it was attributed to testing. South Korea also created about 50 drive-through testing centers and tested many more than any other country very quickly. They treated and isolated infected individuals right away.

South Korea was hailed (justifiably so) as The Flash in acting nimble and fast in their response to SARS-CoV-2. It is interesting that far eastern countries like South Korea, Japan and the Philippines were among the lowest in per capita fatalities compared to western countries. Obesity has to be one distinguishing reason.

In April 2020, Google and Apple announced plans to be able to, at the user's option, track and monitor locations of infected people. To Americans that sounded very Orwellian, but South Korea did just that to help mitigate the spread. South Korea was, along with Japan, one of the great successes in minimizing the impact of COVID-19.

Below are the case and death totals for South Korea in early June.

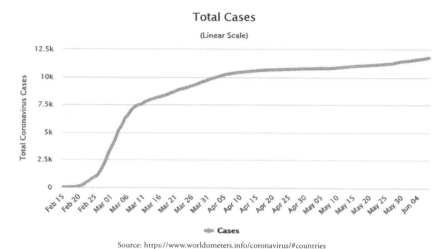

Source: https://www.worldometers.info/coronavirus/#countries

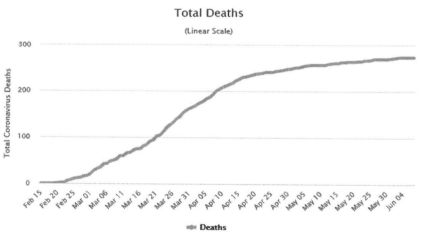

Source: https://www.worldometers.info/coronavirus/#countries

IRAN

Iran issued a complete lockdown on March 27, centered around disciplined social distancing. Iran ended up with a briefer lockdown than most countries. Some reported this was because the government leaders could not agree on what to do, or because a handful had contracted the virus and were out of work a few days. For a hard-hit country, Iran had one of the lighter lockdown measures.

Below are the case and death totals for Iran in early June.

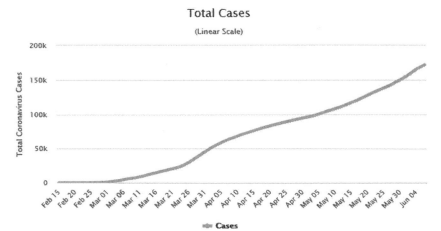

Total Cases
(Linear Scale)

Source: https://www.worldometers.info/coronavirus/#countries

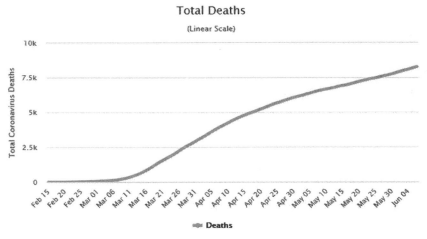

Total Deaths
(Linear Scale)

Source: https://www.worldometers.info/coronavirus/#countries

ICELAND

At a glance you may think Iceland is so remote they may be insulated from a pandemic; this island country of 365,000 people is hundreds of miles from Europe and Greenland. Iceland did close its borders but exercised a much more interesting approach to minimizing the spread of the virus.

Hafsteinn Dan Kristjánsson wrote a great article about it in *Verfassungsblog*. Iceland gave "recommendations or advices and providing information. Among the recommendations repeated over and over again is washing and sanitizing hands, avoid touching, adhering to the two-meter rule wherever possible and to self-isolate or quarantine in certain situations. These are not hard and fast legal rules backed up with sanctions. This is the rule of common sense."[87]

There are downsides of course. You're probably thinking some degree of anarchy may set in, people not following the rules. Fortunately, in a small community like that with like-minded occupants, getting people to play along would be like getting Alaska to play along. But without great population density (8 people per square mile; New York City is 27,000 people per square mile), social distancing is inherent to living in Iceland.

Iceland, with a small population to manage and analyze, by mid-April 2020 tested 6% of its population for COVID-19, very high results at this point for any country. Around 43% of the people testing positive were not symptomatic.

Below are the case and death totals for Iceland in in early June:

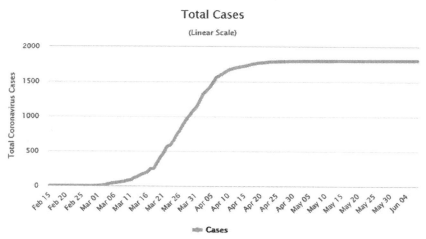

Source: https://www.worldometers.info/coronavirus/#countries

Total Deaths

(Linear Scale)

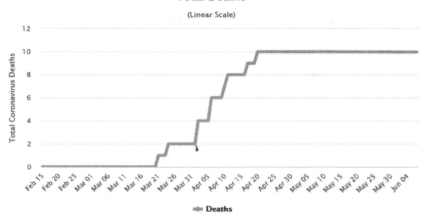

Source: https://www.worldometers.info/coronavirus/#countries

INDIA

India, with a population of 1.3B people and a very low elderly population, locked down their already-fragile economy on March 25. With four hours' notice, Indians were instructed to not leave their homes for an initially set twenty-one days. At the time of the lockdown, India had about five hundred cases of SARS-CoV-2, an incredible step to take given the low positive test number.

India has a huge population of manual labor, small vendor and unincorporated or non-government workers that, when forced to work from home, would not be able to work at all. Estimates are that more than 90% of the population falls into this category – far-exceeding one billion people. When you write those sentences out, you feel an emptiness in your stomach over how challenging people in other countries have it compared to Americans.

Essential businesses like food shops, banks and gas stations remained open. Two questions had to haunt Indians: how do you maintain social distancing in such densely populated areas, and always a vital need for anyone, where do you get the money to survive if you can't get out and work? "*This situation is worse than war,*" said Arun Kumar, an economics professor at the Institute of Social Sciences in New Delhi. "*If we are not able to provide essentials to the bottom 50 percent of the population, then there will be social revolt.*"[88]

Below is a SARS-CoV-2 progression of India's positive tests (cases) for the period beginning and through their lockdown. Their case chart for the lockdown period is over the page:

Total Cases

(Linear Scale)

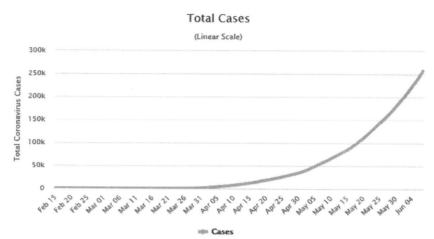

Source: https://www.worldometers.info/coronavirus/#countries

Below a their chart of India deaths for the same period. This total was about the same as Massachusetts at the same time.

Total Deaths

(Linear Scale)

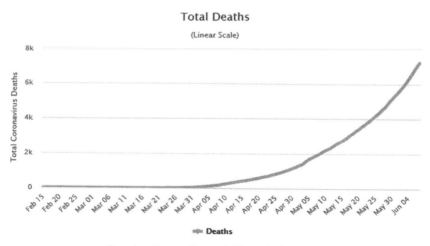

Source: https://www.worldometers.info/coronavirus/#countries

Based on the case studies from the cruise ships and knowing that less any outliers, the only vulnerable group are the elderly (very few as a percent of India's population) or those with underlying health conditions, why would they do this? One of my neighbors has many family members in India and immediately pondered if a revolution was imminent. India has one of the youngest populations in the world and just about the lowest obesity rate in the world. No demographic data would stack up to support that SARS-CoV-2 would ravage Indians justifying the economic ruin.

India had one of the lowest deaths per million at 7 by mid-June, an incredible number assuming the data is accurate, questioning why they would lock down so severely.

CHAPTER 9

LOCKDOWN

On December 3, 1979, The Who performed a concert in Cincinnati, Ohio at a downtown arena similar to today's basketball arenas. Just a young boy at the time, I had listened to the album they were promoting, *Who Are You*, on an eight-track cassette, until the tape got tangled up in the player. The Who was then one of the biggest musical draws in the world. They sold general admission tickets to this concert.

The doors were supposed to open at 3 p.m. but did not open until after 7 p.m. One set of doors opened earlier than the others and fans from the back began pushing forward to get in. Eventually, the push into the funnel of two open doors crushed fans and 11 died of asphyxiation. An uncontrollable flood can break any system. That would not happen at a concert again. I later saw The Who through general admission access at the Pontiac Silverdome (80,000+ fans) and entry was smooth.

With the panic-inducing Imperial College model seeming hauntingly real, the United States and governments across the world were faced with challenging options. With no vaccine in hand and sure-thing treatments still unknown, what do you do? The panic by mid-March was what would happen if all the hospitals and ICUs were slammed at the same time. As we saw in the models, worst case at the peak of the then-respected Imperial College model was a nine-fold shortfall.

WHY WE LOCKED DOWN

The purpose of a lockdown is not to stop the virus spread (though ideal if possible). The purpose is to slow it down so the hospitalizations did not exceed capacity, like preventing the fan rush at the Cincinnati Who concert. The puzzling thing after observing the data from the cruise ships was that it seemed illogical that there would be such an outbreak of hospitalizations or realized COVID-19 deaths. By mid-April hospitals were going broke from their inability to serve non-COVID-19 patients and the lack of COVID-19 patients.

The insanity reached a new level in American history in late April. Hospitals were not overwhelmed. In fact, they never reached capacity with COVID-19 patients. As hospitals stayed empty, were going broke, the curve was flat, states remained closed as unemployment claims reached forty million. Forty million. It's a hard number to grasp, but that is about 20% of the workforce.

The curve was moving downward in hospitalizations, the number that matters. Cases going up were a good sign as hospitalizations did not, validating the virus is not as lethal as once thought. Meanwhile, most in the media were championing continued lockdowns without ever presenting critical data analysis. It became a circular argument: polls supported lockdowns because of the media hype, and the media hype perpetuated the lockdown argument.

On March 11, my son traveled with his college baseball team to California for a weekend series. By the morning of March 12, they announced the game that evening would be played in front of no fans. By late afternoon they canceled the weekend series. By the evening of March 13, the Big-12 season was cancelled, and he was coming home to finish up the semester online and at home. It was still unclear exactly how this would impact us in America, and if so, how bad it was going to get.

The NBA suspended their season on March 11. The NCAA tournament was canceled on March 12, disappointing for this Michigan State alumni. On March 14, Vail Resorts closed most of their ski resorts, which is most of the ski resorts in America, due to SARS-CoV-2 fears. On March 17, The Rolling Stones canceled their spring tour in America.

The summer Olympics, the French Open, the Kentucky Derby, the NHL, the PGA Tour, Major League Baseball, everything was cancelled or postponed. Americans were not yet in a lockdown nor had they experienced any real health impacts as it thundered in with an emptiness of an impending new reality.

On March 11, 2020, President Trump declared that all flights to and from 26 countries in Europe would cease. Those countries included: Austria, Belgium, Czech Republic, Denmark, Estonia, Finland, France, Germany, Greece, Hungary, Iceland, Italy, Latvia, Liechtenstein, Lithuania, Luxembourg, Malta, Netherlands, Norway, Poland, Portugal, Slovakia, Slovenia, Spain, Sweden, and Switzerland.[89] The United Kingdom was added days later.

Before official lockdowns by state, city or county were rolled out, many businesses took the cue from the travel bans and fear of an outbreak and took their own preventive measures. Retailers began temporary closing stores. By March 20, Nike, Patagonia, Neiman Marcus, The Gap and hundreds of shopping malls closed. Grocery store inventory was washed out from the sea of shoppers stocking up. The unusual item in short supply? Toilet paper. It became a quarantine hot commodity and sales doubled year over year in March. Hopefully savvy investors got out of airline stocks and into Procter and Gamble or Kimberly Clark in time. P&G stock cratered like many stocks but jumped 30% within 30 days, as did Kimberly Clark.

THE FIRST LOCKDOWN: CALIFORNIA

California became the first state to lockdown on March 20, 2020. In late April, the CDC confirmed the first two COVID-19 deaths in the United States were in Santa Clara, CA on February 17. Illinois and New York followed immediately. It was a surreal headline to digest. California. Forty million people. The largest state economy in the United States. On its own, the fifth largest economy in the world, was shut down. This had to be the hardest and most consequential decision California Governor Gavin Newsom would make in his life.

The official order:

EXECUTIVE DEPARTMENT STATE OF CALIFORNIA

EXECUTIVE ORDER N-33-20

WHEREAS on March 4, 2020, I proclaimed a State of Emergency to exist in California as a result of the threat of COVID-19; and

WHEREAS in a short period of time, COVID-19 has rapidly spread throughout California, necessitating updated and more stringent guidance from federal, state, and local public health officials; and

WHEREAS for the preservation of public health and safety throughout the entire State of California, I find it necessary for all Californians to heed the State public health directives from the Department of Public Health.

NOW, THEREFORE, I, GAVIN NEWSOM, Governor of the State of California, in accordance with the authority vested in me by the State Constitution and statutes of the State of California, and in particular, Government Code sections 8567, 8627, and 8665 do hereby issue the following Order to become effective immediately:

IT IS HEREBY ORDERED THAT:

1) To preserve the public health and safety, and to ensure the healthcare delivery system is capable of serving all, and prioritizing those at the highest risk and vulnerability, all residents are directed to immediately heed the current State public health directives, which I ordered the Department of Public Health to develop for the current statewide status of COVID-19. Those directives are consistent with the March 19, 2020, Memorandum on Identification of Essential Critical Infrastructure Workers During COVID-19 Response, found at: https://covid 19.ca.gov/. Those directives follow:

ORDER OF THE STATE PUBLIC HEALTH OFFICER March 19, 2020

To protect public health, I as State Public Health Officer and Director of the California Department of Public Health order all individuals living in the State of California to stay home or at their place of residence except as needed to maintain continuity of operations of the federal critical infrastructure sectors, as outlined at https://www.cisa.gov/identifying-critical-infrastructure-during-covid-19. In addition, and in consultation with the Director of the Governor's Office of Emergency Services, I may designate additional sectors as critical in order to protect the health and well-being of all Californians.

Pursuant to the authority under the Health and Safety Code 120125, 120140, 131080, 120130(c), 120135, 120145, 120175 and 120150, this order is to go into effect immediately and shall stay in effect until further notice.

The federal government has identified 16 critical infrastructure sectors whose assets, systems, and networks, whether physical or virtual, are considered so vital to the United States that their incapacitation or destruction would have a debilitating effect on security, economic security, public health or safety, or any combination thereof. I order that Californians working in these 16 critical infrastructure sectors may continue their work because of the importance of these sectors to Californians' health and well-being. This Order is being issued to protect the public health of Californians. The California Department of Public Health looks to establish consistency across the state in order to ensure that we mitigate the impact of COVID-19. Our goal is simple, we want to bend the curve, and disrupt the spread of the virus. The supply chain must continue, and Californians must have access to such necessities as food, prescriptions, and health care. When people need to leave their homes or places of residence, whether to obtain or perform the functions above, or to otherwise facilitate authorized necessary activities, they should at all times practice social distancing. 2) The healthcare delivery system shall prioritize services to serving those who are the sickest and shall prioritize resources, including personal protective equipment, for the providers providing direct care to them. 3) The Office of Emergency Services is directed to take necessary steps to ensure compliance with this Order. 4) This Order shall be enforceable pursuant to California law, including, but not limited to, Government Code section 8665. IT IS FURTHER ORDERED that as soon as hereafter possible, this Order be filed in the Office of the Secretary of State and that widespread publicity and notice be given of this Order. This Order is not intended to, and does not, create any rights or benefits, substantive or procedural, enforceable at law or in equity, against the State of California, its agencies, departments, entities, officers, employees, or any other person.

The sixteen critical infrastructure sectors were: chemical, commercial facilities, communications, critical manufacturing, dams, defense industrial base, emergency services, energy, financial service, food and agriculture, government facilities, health care and public health, information technology, nuclear reactors, materials and waste, transportation systems and water and wastewater systems.

Many businesses and employees fit in these broad sector classifications, but there was no doubt which businesses were on temporary leave: dine-in restaurants, bars and clubs, gyms, any entertainment venues, any public gatherings, clothing retailers (other than superstores like Walmart, Target, etc.). Schools were closed and childcare became a challenge for many parents, whether they were confined to their homes or not.

At the time of Governor Newsom's order, California had 699 confirmed cases of SARS-CoV-2 and suggested 55% of the state would become infected within eight weeks. Around 14% of California's population is over 65.

California hospitals were working to increase their capacity another 40% providing 30,000 additional beds. On April 16, of California's 80,939 hospital beds and 6,986 ICUs, 3,324 COVID-19 patients were hospitalized and of them, 1,184 ended up in ICUs. On May 7, 3,319 were hospitalized, flat from three weeks prior, and 3,302 people were lost to COVID-19 by May 18.[90]

In mid-May, California was below expectations in all deaths compared to the previous three-year average. To repeat, all-cause deaths were below average year to date in the midst of the lockdown. In late June California was 2% above the all-cause death average year to date.

Based on the 55% infection rate suggested (which would surely be lower the older you get because elderly circulate less than younger people – public transportation, working, going out, traveling), of the 5.6MM people over 65 years old, 3.1MM would get infected. Based on the rates taken from the two cruise ships, it's hard to imagine a total hospitalization of more than 125,000 for the total time period. Considering the gradual distribution of hospitalizations, it would be nearly impossible for California to reach capacity with COVID-19 patients. California ended the spring realizing better fatality rates than even the cruise ships.

On April 2, one of the more interesting violators of the stay at home order was arrested, demonstrating the ridiculousness of these orders and police-state some were heading. A young man was seen paddle-boarding off Malibu Beach and was reported. The Lost Hills Sheriff's office was called and the man was pursued until he came to shore. The man was arrested for Disobeying a Lifeguard 17.12.115 LACC and Violation of Government Code 8665. The suspect was transported to Lost Hills Sheriff's Station where he was booked and released on a promise to appear.

He was arrested and booked and faced up to a $1,000 fine and or up to six months in jail. How far would the state go to enforce this law while others could access hiking trails while keeping social distance? Meanwhile, California released 3,500 nonviolent inmates within the next 60 days, and New York City had released 900 people as of March 31. As states were releasing convicted criminals serving time, this surfer was arrested for getting some time in the outdoors by himself.

On April 10, Riverside County launched an app that could be downloaded from the Apple Store or Google Play for residents to report on stay-at-home violations. Users could upload a picture of the violation and the idea was that law enforcement would pursue the perpetrators.[91]

By early May, COVID-19 deaths were on a steep decline, and hospitals were ghost towns. Los Angeles Mayor Eric Garcetti and politicians nationally forgot the reason we shut down communities in the first place was not to stop the spread of the virus as a primary objective, but to slow it down so hospital capacity would not be overwhelmed.

With deaths declining and hospitals empty, for some reason politicians kept talking about locking down while little was happening.

Californians protested as the lockdowns persisted against any real health crisis reaching hospitals, with California one of the lowest per capita impacted states in the country. As other states reopened in early May, and California barely budged, the sheriff in Riverside County, east of Los Angeles with more than two million people, said his office would stop enforcing lockdowns on businesses and people. Holes were appearing in the dike.

OTHER STATES FOLLOW CALIFORNIA

California locking down sent shockwaves through the country. The largest state in the country taking an extreme measure sent a message to other states that this was an appropriate policy and there would be little political pressure, media pressure or even public outcry. Plus, in mid-March, no one really knew what would happen with SARS-CoV-2. These shutdowns were the most consequential domestic economic policy decision in American history.

Not every state shut down, however. Five of the fifty states did not have a shelter-in-place policy: Arkansas, Iowa, South Dakota, North Dakota and Nebraska. Details on select state's orders and COVID-19 hospitalizations, deaths, and healthcare capacity are listed below:

ALABAMA

Governor Kay Ivey issued a stay at home order a week after closing all "non-essential businesses." Initially, Ivey tried to put in place some limitations without limiting personal travel though schools, beaches, gyms, personal care providers, and dine-in restaurants closed. There was no statewide quarantine. Functionally, this would be similar to most states. Alabama realized 1,188 total hospitalizations and 369 deaths by early May 2020. Alabama has 15,000 hospital beds and 1,097 ICU beds in the state.[92]

ALASKA

Alaska went on a lighter lockdown than some states. Traveling was limited to essential needs, gatherings of less than ten people, and nonessential businesses limited to minimum operations or remote work. Travelers from out of state were to quarantine for 14 days. Restaurants were to be limited to takeout. Native Alaskan communities are often very remote, with access only by flying in and out. They also put strict guidelines in place, mostly on who could come in and out. It's easy to envision these tight communities trying to keep outsiders out while SARS-CoV-2 was spreading. Alaska had 38 hospitalizations and 10 deaths by early May 2020 with a capacity of 1,658 hospital beds and 106 ICU beds.[93]

ARIZONA

While not exercising a statewide quarantine, Arizona followed most states in orders other than not locking down parks unless local authorities do so.[94] By the end of April, Arizona had 1,449 people hospitalized with COVID-19 and 450 fatalities. Arizona has 13,296 hospital beds and 1,302 ICU Beds. Arizona remained shut down even with this data released. In late June Arizona did hit their high of cases and hospitalizations, though many were classified as "suspected." It's not clear what prompted this spike, though they along with other southern states experienced similar.

ARKANSAS

Arkansas was one of the five "lighter shutdown" states, though Governor Asa Hutchinson closed personal care shops, eat-in portions of restaurants and gyms. Some malls remained open, though within that many stores opted to close. Food courts were closed as were children's play areas. Arkansas reported 466 COVID-19 patients hospitalized through early May with 93 on a ventilator, and 88 deaths.[95] Arkansas has a total of 9,041 hospital beds and 640 ICU beds.[96]

COLORADO

Before the state locked down, on March 14, Vail Resorts shut down their vast number of ski resorts, shocking spring breakers and sending a chill of reality of what may happen all over soon. As a recreational climber, it was good to see the 14ers open for hiking. Colorado's order was largely the same as the other states, also allowing for the opening of hardware stores, marijuana stores, and keeping parks open but requiring a safe distance. By May 7, Colorado had 2,123 COVID-19 patients hospitalized since mid-March and counted 944 fatalities by May 7 (a number that would fluctuate later in May). Colorado has 9,955 hospital beds and 885 ICUs.[97]

One of the craziest lockdown violation stories came out of Colorado on April 7, 2020. A former Colorado State Patrol Trooper was playing t-ball with his six-year-old daughter at a near empty softball field. This struck a chord with me because baseball was our family life for a decade, and at my son's same age we were at fields practicing a good four days a week. He was instructed by police on the scene to leave and that the park was closed, even though it was open. The police arrested him in front of his daughter, releasing him not long after at the scene.

Never mind that the police were wrong about the park being closed, this really demonstrated an overreach in actual application and the spirit of the law. In reality, Colorado was in no crisis. A man was getting outdoors with his daughter. Hoping this would help illuminate the absurdity of the lockdowns, nothing really changed.

CONNECTICUT

Connecticut, close to New York City and with many residents working in the city, experienced a much higher than average COVID-19 impact. On April 22, 2020, Connecticut had 1,949 patients hospitalized with COVID-19, just past its peak and a total of 2,797 fatalities by May 7.[98] Connecticut ended up with the third highest number of deaths per capita by mid-June. Connecticut has 8,805 hospital beds and 594 ICUs.

FLORIDA

Florida's lockdown order required 14-day quarantining for visitors from the New York/New Jersey/Connecticut tri-state area. On May 7, Florida had 6,765 total hospitalizations and 1,600 fatalities. Florida has 56,039 hospital beds and 4,787 ICUs. With a higher than average number of elderly residents and close ties to the tri-state area, one would expect Florida to have a high contribution to the COVID-19 hospitalizations and deaths. Florida did not permit incoming drivers from Louisiana for a few weeks.[99]

Florida was later than some states to lock down and made headlines when beaches were open during spring break in March. *Business Insider* ran this headline at the time: "Florida's spring break problem shows a political pandemic divide: Red and blue states are treating coronavirus differently." That played out true as

April and May unfolded. Governor Ron DeSantis did not order early beach closings, and mayors in towns in Broward and Dade counties closed their beaches sooner than those in St. Petersburg. Making much bigger headlines was Jacksonville's Mayor Lenny Curry when he reopened the beaches there on April 17, 2020.

Critics started a Twitter hashtag *#FloridaMorons* and it began trending. Mainstream media outlets crucified the mayor for the decision, led by headlines like this from *The Washington Post:* "In Florida, we love our beaches. Thanks to our governor, now we can die for them" by Diane Roberts, a journalist and professor of English at Florida State University. In the article, Roberts slammed Governor DeSantis and President Trump, largely with the claim that "how can we open the beaches until we know how many people have [SARS-CoV-2]?" With hospitals empty, when do you open the beaches? Would Roberts suggest they wait until next April?

GEORGIA

Georgia followed similar orders as most states and did not make headlines until Governor Brian Kemp announced the state would begin opening up on Friday, April 24. *Vox* ran a piece critical of the decision, writing this: "The coronavirus crisis is hardly over in Georgia, but the state's leadership has decided it's time to start reopening parts of the economy there anyway. Republican Gov. Kemp announced in a tweet on Monday that businesses such as gyms, hair salons, barbershops, tattoo parlors, bowling alleys, and nail salons will be allowed to resume some operations on Friday, April 24."

By May 7, Georgia had 5,866 total hospitalizations, 1,384 ICU admissions and 1,352 fatalities attributed to COVID-19. Georgia has 24,135 hospital beds and 2,223 ICUs.[100] Their death total doubled by late June but at a lower rate than the beginning of the pandemic and after reopening.

HAWAII

Hawaii continued their March lockdown order through May 31. Hawaii issued a mandatory stay-at-home lockdown order and 14-day travel quarantine with strict limitations on outdoor activities. Governor David Ige took a particularly strong stance on the lockdown, imposing a mandatory 14-day stay-at-home order, banning nonessential foot and vehicle traffic after 4:30 p.m. Did you know the coronavirus spreads more aggressively after 4:30 p.m. than before?

Violators may be punished by fines of up to $5,000 and a year in jail. In March, the Honolulu police issued 70 citations and arrested two. On Kauai, police set up checkpoints. Restaurants were closed, no loitering on the beach or exercising, and walking outside required social distancing. Did the governor know

SARS-CoV-2 wasn't spreading outdoors? Hawaii has 3,189 hospital beds and 189 ICUs. By May 7, Hawaii had 74 total hospitalizations and 17 deaths.[101]

ILLINOIS

Home to America's third largest city, Chicago, Illinois was one of the first states to lock down. Illinois's lockdown order did not require a quarantine but closed the same as most other states, including the state parks and outdoor recreational areas. As of May 7, Illinois reported 4,877 hospital beds and 1,253 ventilators cumulatively used for COVID-19 cases, and 3,111 deaths. Illinois has 31,876 total hospital beds, 3,695 ICUs and over 3,000 ventilators.[102]

Incredibly, on April 23, 2020, Governor JB Pritzker extended the stay-at-home issue through the end of May, even though they were not near hospital capacity at that time. Hospitalizations were declining, and everyone knew by then that only the most vulnerable (elderly and those with certain comorbidities) were likely to be affected. Meanwhile, by late April, Illinois had more than 750,000 unemployment claims in five weeks. Why wouldn't the state unlock their economy while ensuring the vulnerable were protected? We will see why when analyzing the media and politics hanging over the pandemic in a coming chapter.

On May 13, Peoria County announced they would ignore the governor's order and begin the end of the shutdown order. Madison County, in a 26-2 county board vote, joined to reopen and eight other counties downstate joined in.

IOWA

Governor Kim Reynolds did not order a shelter-in-place and even made the comment that health care officials like Dr. Anthony Fauci "can't just look at a map" and make such demands. Nonessential businesses were closed but parks remained open and no one was quarantined. She sent the image below demonstrating trust in Iowans to act responsibly. On May 7, Iowa had a total of 417 COVID-19 hospitalizations and 231 deaths. Iowa has 9,126 hospital beds available and 416 ICUs.[103]

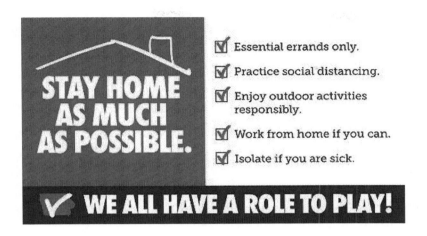

KANSAS

Kansas quarantined their residents who traveled to California, Florida, New York or Washington state after March 14, or visited Illinois or New Jersey after March 22, for 14 days, or who had close contact with a Covid-19 patient. On May 7, Kansas cumulatively had 547 hospitalizations and 165 deaths. Kansas has 9,242 hospital beds in total and 627 ICUs.[104]

KENTUCKY

Similar to most states, Kentucky issued a stay-at-home order with a couple exceptions: anyone coming in from out of state—including residents—must self-quarantine for 14 days upon return, and state parks are closed for overnight stays.[105]

Kentucky made headlines around Easter services on April 12, 2020. Kentucky Governor Andy Beshear issued a warning that anyone violating the state's stay-at-home order was subject to a 14-day mandatory self-quarantine, going on to say that the state will record license plate information of people seen attending mass gatherings and turn that information over to local public health officials. Quarantine notices were then delivered in person. This warning sparked controversy between supporters of the policy and those feeling like attending service on the most important Christian holiday via a drive-in was government overreach.

Kentucky Senator Rand Paul tweeted this on Twitter in response: *"Taking license plates at church? Quarantining someone for being Christian on Easter Sunday? Someone needs to take a step back here."* On Fire Christian Church sued Louisville Mayor Greg Fischer and the city after Fischer prepared to enforce the governor's order. U.S. District Judge Justin Walker sided with the church, saying that the city is prohibited from *"enforcing; attempting to enforce; threatening to enforce; or otherwise requiring compliance with any prohibition on drive-in church services at On Fire."*

Kentucky had 1,519 total hospitalizations and 597 ICU patients by May 7, and 294 deaths due to COVID-19. Kentucky has 14,022 total hospital beds and 1,259 ICUs.

LOUISIANA

Louisiana shut down with travel outside the home for necessary needs, but no quarantine. Gatherings were limited to ten people, and some parks remained open for fishing, hiking, and biking outdoors. New Orleans was hit harder than any area after the New York City area and Detroit.

New Orleans's most famous tradition is Mardi Gras, and in 2020 it occurred on February 25th. A typical Mardi Gras attracts approximately 1.4 million people, and if you've seen pictures, everyone is close. While "social distancing" of six feet is up for debate, the circulation at Mardi Gras is more akin to a traveling through New York's subways at rush hour. The first case of COVID-19 was reported on March 9, and the first victim was at Mardi Gras. Whether Mardi Gras was the catalyst for the quick outbreak is strong speculation.

On March 13, Governor John Bel Edwards closed the schools and prohibited all gatherings of more than 250 people. On March 15, that first-case patient died. On April 9, Louisiana had 2,054 patients in hospitals. They reported 2,135 fatalities and as the curve was bending downward by May 7, they would have 1,432 COVID-19 patients in hospitals. Louisiana has a total of 14,977 hospital beds and 1,215 ICUs. Louisiana also appears to have the highest ratio of hospitalizations to fatalities, perhaps because many residents suffer from obesity, diabetes and high blood pressure.

According to the Louisiana Department of Health, of the COVID-19 fatalities, the victims had the following underlying conditions.[106] They are not mutually exclusive; some patients would have a combination of conditions:

- Asthma – 3.94%
- Cancer – 7.66%
- Cardiac disease – 18.56%
- Chronic kidney disease – 20.11%
- Congestive heart failure – 10.36%
- Diabetes – 34.73%
- Hypertension – 56.15%
- Neurological – 7.42%
- Obesity – 19.72%
- Pulmonary – 11.76

MAINE

Travelers arriving in Maine, regardless of their state of residency, were required to self-quarantine for 14 days. Maine has 3,408 hospital beds and would experience 51 COVID-19 deaths by the end of April.[107]

With hospital beds empty, the curve turning downward, and a fatality rate of COVID-19 at 0.0039% against their total population, on April 28, Governor Janet Mills extended their stay-at-home order through May, while states like Texas and Florida were opening up that same day. Social gatherings of more than 10 people remained prohibited, and visitors from out of state were still required to self-quarantine.[108]

MARYLAND

Maryland had a similar shut down order to Maine, closed their beaches but left some parks open. On May 7, Maryland had 1,683 COVID-19 hospitalizations, half of its peak, and suffered 1,410 deaths. Maryland has 10,977 hospital beds and 962 ICUs. The chart below gives you a visual of the total hospital beds available at the top and the actual COVID-19 capacity and ventilator capacity below it.[109]

ICU and Acute Hospital Beds for COVID-19, Currently in Use

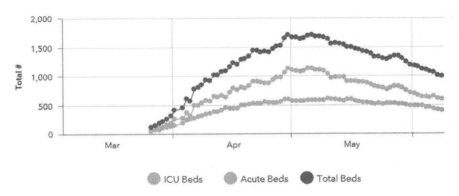

MASSACHUSETTS

Massachusetts employed a similar shut down policy as Maine. While 4,552 people lost their lives attributed to COVID-19 through May 7, and 7,235 were hospitalized, we will see later that some of those suspected deaths due to the virus are not all verified. Massachusetts has 15,150 hospital beds and 1,273 ICUs.[110] By May, 61% of all deaths were sourced from within nursing homes.

MICHIGAN

Michigan became the second epicenter of the COVID-19 epidemic for three reasons: a significant outbreak in Detroit, high profile actions and statements by Governor Gretchen Whitmer and protests against the lockdowns in April and May. Growing up in the Detroit area, attending college at Michigan State University, and traveling there several times a year to see family always keeps me following Michigan happenings. My brother is a surgeon in Michigan and my mother and her husband live in the city of Detroit. Michigan moved into swing-state status after President Trump won that state in 2016.

Detroit, once the second largest city in America, is the heart of the auto industry, with General Motors, Ford and Chrysler headquartered there. After the civil rights riots in the summer of 1967, Detroit experienced "white flight," where a majority of white residents left the city limits for the suburbs in Oakland and Macomb counties. Detroit sits in Wayne County. The Detroit Tigers winning the 1968 World Series is often credited with bringing unity back to the city.

Beyond the Detroit metropolitan area, most of Michigan is made up of college towns and smaller communities. Fishing and hunting are very popular in Michigan. The Great Lakes surround Michigan as well as thousands of inland lakes, with Canadian borders to the north and east across the lakes. Michigan has been one of the hardest-hit states in unemployment and underemployment as the auto industry shifted to more automation (thus fewer manufacturing jobs) and plants moving to Mexico due to much lower labor costs.

Michigan counted 4,313 lives lost to COVID-19 by May 7 and about 6,000 in late June. Most had underlying conditions, as 90%-plus of all Americans hospitalized for COVID-19 did. At the peak of the pandemic, 3,826 patients were hospitalized at once, 1,628 in critical care and 1,434 on ventilators.[111] Michigan has 24,649 hospital beds and 1,894 ICUs in the state. The chart on the next page illustrates the trend down from their peak in overall hospitalizations and those in an ICU and on a ventilator.

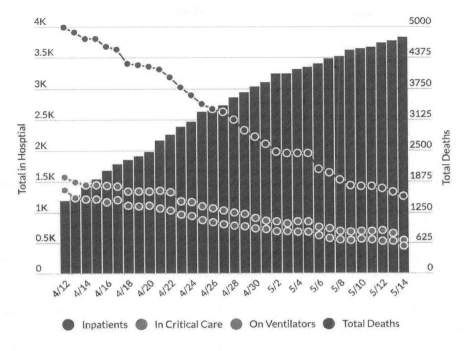

LOCKDOWN

Inpatients ● In Critical Care ● On Ventilators ● Total Deaths

Source: https://www.clickondetroit.com/news/local/2020/05/16/tracking-michigan-covid-19-hospitalization-data-trends/

The chart below illustrates how hard Michigan was impacted in absolute numbers of deaths compared to neighboring states, with Illinois and Ohio each more populated than Michigan.

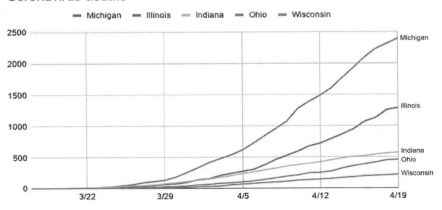

Coronavirus deaths

— Michigan — Illinois — Indiana — Ohio — Wisconsin

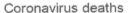

WHO DIED IN MICHIGAN

Some media personalities called out issues associated with racism because more than 50% of Michigan's COVID-19 victims were black. Peeling this back, in 2020 85% of Detroit was comprised of black residents. Most Detroit residents are ridiculously poor, you will see evidence of blight on any drive in the city off Woodward Avenue. With the city the epicenter of the outbreak in the state, and black residents having a higher-than-average propensity for obesity, diabetes, heart disease and other chronic lung disorders, it was a sad perfect storm affecting Detroit residents. Wayne County was not the only county stressed in Michigan. Oakland County and Macomb County are next to Detroit's Wayne County, predominately white, and each were impacted similarly to Wayne County in cases, hospitalizations and fatalities.[112]

In speaking with doctors and medical staff in Detroit, they found themselves overwhelmed for that same three-week period. They are used to taking care of patients with influenza-related illness. While many of these patients ultimately die, their course is one of gradual clinical deterioration. Conversely, COVID-19 patients could be clinically stable, only to see their condition rapidly deteriorate in a matter of hours. An anesthesiologist who was intubating patients with respiratory failure told me he thought to himself *"I may be the last person this patient ever sees."*

A seasoned nurse anesthetist worked a 24-hour shift in which she had to intubate several COVID patients. She was called to intubate a patient with respiratory distress, but he refused to be intubated. This may have been due to fear resulting from multiple early reports stating that virtually all patients who were intubated went on to die. She subsequently told me that she hoped never to have another shift like that.

WHY MICHIGAN?

Why was Michigan hit so hard? It appears a few things may have all contributed to this.[113] First, in early February, Detroit Metro Airport was one of 11 airports where incoming travelers from China were diverted for screenings and or quarantines. With the auto industry based in Detroit and with manufacturing ties to China, travelers may have carried SARS-CoV-2 into the area through several different points.

The city of Detroit is reliant on public transportation, and while not densely populated like New York, it is more than many other cities.

POLITICS AND COVID-19 IN MICHIGAN

On March 10, Governor Whitmer said this when she issued an order to lockdown the state: "*The main goal of these efforts is to slow the spread of the virus, not to stop it. It has moved into Michigan.*"

Controversy soon swirled in Michigan. Joe Biden had announced in a debate leading up to Super Tuesday that he would, if the Democrat nominee, select a female running mate. Immediately short lists were created and debated, and Governor Whitmer emerged on the short list. Whitmer was the Democrat representative to deliver President Trump's state of the union address opposition party response, speaking in East Lansing, Michigan.

Gretchen Whitmer is a lawyer by trade, and with accomplished parents. Her father was the president of Blue Cross Blue Shield of Michigan and her mother was an assistant state attorney general. Whitmer, a graduate of Michigan State University for both undergrad and law school, served as a Michigan state senator.

It started on March 17, 2020, when Whitmer was interviewed on MSNBC and said, "*the federal government did not take this seriously early enough…to hear the leader of the federal government tell us to work around the federal government because it's too slow is kind of mind-boggling, to be honest.*" Her response was referring to a comment President Trump made on March 16, suggesting governors take the lead on securing their own healthcare equipment such as ventilators. Governors are elected to manage their state needs, and playing this out, a governor would identify needs and then fill those needs through the federal government, other states or the private sector.

On March 20, President Trump and team were delivering their daily briefing on the COVID-19 crisis. Those press briefing became lengthy each day. In most press briefings and even at rallies, Trump tends to speak extemporaneously. He offered up that hydroxychloroquine, a malaria treatment drug, might be effective for treating COVID-19. He was criticized sharply by his critics for this, and Dr. Anthony Fauci was less than committal on its benefit. *The Washington Post* referred to his comment as recommending snake oil.[114]

Whitmer reacted swiftly and on March 24, Michigan's Department of Licensing and Regulatory Affairs sent a letter warning health care providers not to prescribe hydroxychloroquine.[115] The letter read:

> "*Prescribing hydroxychloroquine or chloroquine without further proof of efficacy for treating COVID-19 or with the intent to stockpile the drug may create a shortage for patients with lupus, rheumatoid arthritis, or*

other ailments for which chloroquine and hydroxychloroquine are proven treatments. Reports of this conduct will be evaluated and may be further investigated for administrative action. Prescribing any kind of prescription must also be associated with medical documentation showing proof of the medical necessity and medical condition for which the patient is being treated. Again, these are drugs that have not been proven scientifically or medically to treat COVID-19."

This political sparring was taking place center stage in a healthcare crisis where no known sure-thing treatments were known yet.

On April 1, *The New York Times* reported this headline: "A group of moderately ill people were given hydroxychloroquine, which appeared to ease their symptoms quickly, but more research is needed."[116]

On April 2, *The New York Post* wrote this: "Of 2,171 physicians surveyed, 37 percent rated hydroxychloroquine the "most effective therapy" for combating the potentially deadly illness."[117]

On April 2, Whitmer reversed her stance, saying this:

"The fear that a pronouncement at the federal level might create some hoarding was something that we were very concerned about, because we do have Michigan patients that have been prescribed this drug pre-COVID-19 that we wanted to make sure still had access to their medication," she said. "But I think that, as we know, this is a novel virus, and we have to have the mindset that we're going to be willing to explore what possibilities there are in terms of improving testing, in terms of testing for antibodies ... so we know who is immune, [and are] testing drugs and therapies in the process."

Politics were shining brightly as Whitmer was trying to gain points by standing up to President Trump. However, as Whitmer stated above, it is a novel virus. In the midst of a crisis, many patients would try something with a reasonable chance of improving their condition. There was fury all over the world to try new treatments to find the right solution while a vaccine was unavailable.

Karen Whitsett is a Democrat state representative in Michigan from Detroit. She contracted COVID-19 in April. Feeling ill she took hydroxychloroquine to ease her symptoms. She described it as a miracle drug. Whitsett said,

"I really want to say that you have to give this an opportunity. For me, it saved my life. I only can go by what it is that I have gone through and what my story is, and I can't speak for anyone else. So that's not what I'm trying to do here. I'm only speaking for myself. I did have a difficult time, even that day, obtaining the medication because of an order that was put down in my state. And it was on that day so you can imagine how terrified I was that I had to beg and plead and go through a whole lot to try to get the medication. If President Trump had not talked about this it wouldn't have been something that would be accessible for anyone to be able to get right now."

On April 14th, Whitsett personally thanked President Trump and Vice President Pence. On April 25, Detroit's 13th Congressional District Democratic formally censured Whitsett and withheld any future endorsements of the lawmaker for breaking protocol by meeting the president.[118] A censure is when a political party publicly reprimands a politician. The censure states Whitsett "misrepresented the needs and priorities" of Democratic leadership to the president and public."[119] It's the difference between war time politicians and peace time politicians. Politicians from both parties said we were at war with COVID-19, but they believed it when it was convenient, stopping short of war declarations in favor of partisan politics.

Taking a page from the Illinois leadership playbook, Governor Whitmer's husband would, on May 24 claim executive privilege against the lockdown. He requested a marina to put their boat in the water in northern Michigan so they could go boating over Memorial Day weekend. After all the strict lockdown measures, one of the tightest and longest in the country, the First Family demonstrated the rules didn't apply to them. This really shows that these measures were not necessary or mission-critical in the first place.

MINNESOTA

Minnesota's shutdown directive was in line with all other states. Schools closed but essential activities were permissible as well as exercising outdoors. In a move a little more extreme than other states, the Minneapolis Parks and Recreation Board closed beaches and lakes in the Land of Ten Thousand Lakes.

Minnesota's total cumulative hospitalizations on May 7 were 1,459 and by then suffered 508 COVID-19 deaths, 407 from long-term-care facilities, one of the highest in the country. And 80% of Minnesota's deaths were nursing home residents. As lakes and beaches were closed, no policy was in place to protect the known most vulnerable. Minnesota has 14,528 hospital beds and 905 ICUs.

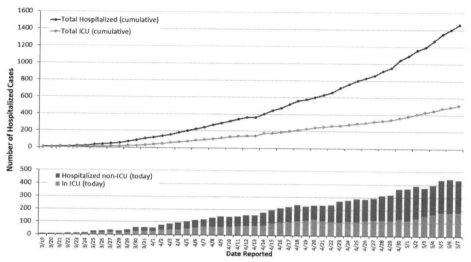

Source: https://www.health.state.mn.us/diseases/coronavirus/situation.html

MISSISSIPPI

Mississippi's shutdown mirrored Alabama's. Mississippi peaked COVID-19 hospital capacity with 401 and lost 396 people by May 7 against a total capacity of 11,785 hospital beds and 633 ICUs. Below is an excellent chart illustrating hospital activity related to COVID-19 provided by the state.

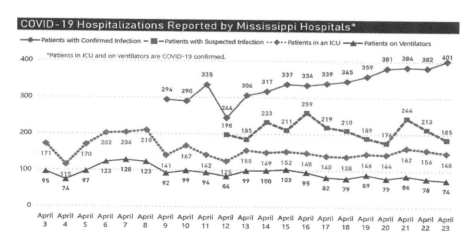

Below is a chart of the underlying conditions of the fatalities in Mississippi. Some would have more than one condition, but you can see nearly all victims had underlying conditions.

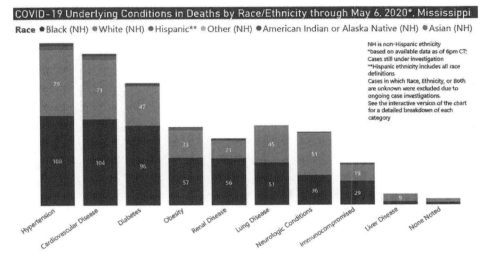

Source: https://msdh.ms.gov/msdhsite/_static/14,0,420.html

NEW JERSEY

New Jersey as an extension of the New York City epicenter suffered one of the worst impacts of COVID-19 in the country. They issued a lockdown measure similar to New York, except only gatherings of more than 10 people were banned. By the time the COVID-19 curve was passed in mid-May, New Jersey had a cumulative hospitalization of 12,946 over a seven-week period. New Jersey has 20,079 hospital beds and 1,670 ICUs. New Jersey would suffer the most deaths to COVID-19 after New York with more than 10,000 by mid-May.

New Jersey's lockdown took an interesting turn on April 18, 2020. New Jersey Governor Phil Murphy shut down people viewing a tulip farm festival, an in-vehicle drive-by activity. Murphy banned gatherings of those with more than 10 people, like most states. That led to some arrests of people violating those orders, claiming they were an infringement of rights. Considering the real crisis hitting the New York area, it is reasonable to understand locking down like they did. However, the tulip-ban took it to a new level.

To put this in some context, New Jersey residents remained able to shop for non-essential items at places like Walmart and Target, interacting pretty much as they had in the past, normal. To ban a drive-through activity like this, particularly when the hospitalizations and deaths were on the sharp decline, brought government overreach to an absurd level.

NORTH DAKOTA

Governor Doug Burgum implemented one of the least intrusive issues of any state in the union. Bars and restaurants were limited to takeout only, and some personal-care (hair stylist businesses, for example) and recreational facilities were closed. Otherwise, much was left open and statewide gatherings were not banned. North Dakota did quarantine travelers coming in from overseas, people traveling from some vacation spots and later Minnesota. Outdoor activities were still allowed, such as hiking, driving to parks and hunting. Walleye fishing was still open, something my brother and I would appreciate. By mid-May, North Dakota realized 102 total COVID-19 hospitalizations and 31 deaths. North Dakota has 3,232 hospital beds and 168 ICUs.[120]

OHIO

Ohio issued similar nonessential business shutdowns, limited travel for essential needs, limited gatherings to 10 people, and kept wildlife areas open. People traveling from out of state were to self-quarantine for 14 days. Ohio eased restrictions on May 1, allowing for non-COVID-related elective medical procedures to be done. They allowed most things to open by May 21, except gyms and similar businesses, albeit with capacity restrictions.

On May 11, Ohio Department of Health Director Dr. Amy Acton shared that six COVID-19 cases were traced back to January. That marked some of the earliest cases known in the country, and far from either coast.

Ohio had 4,140 total COVID-19 hospitalizations by May 7 and 1,271 fatalities, doubling that into late June. Ohio has 31,161 hospital beds and 2,490 ICUs in the state.[121]

OREGON

Governor Kate Brown issued a statewide stay-at-home order on March 23 after having closed schools on March 11. There was not a statewide order issued for any quarantines. All other lockdown measures were about the same as other states. State parks were closed. On May 8, a cumulative total of 596 people were hospitalized for COVID-19 and 121 people lost their lives. Oregon has 6,683 hospital beds and 651 ICUs.

PENNSYLVANIA

Pennsylvania did not quarantine their residents but did limit travel to essential needs. Gatherings were loosely prohibited, and outdoor activities were limited to "passive and dispersed recreation." Governor Tom Wolf announced on April 23 that the state would begin opening up on May 8 in a tiered manner beginning in lower populated areas, with construction work to resume on May 1.

Sixty-eight percent of deaths in Pennsylvania were nursing home residents. Stopping activities, closing stores, people unable to work didn't save them. On March 18, 2020, Pennsylvania required nursing homes to accept COVID-19 admissions, stating:

> *"Nursing care facilities must continue to accept new admissions and receive readmissions for current residents who have been discharged from the hospital who are stable to alleviate the increasing burden in the acute care settings. This may include stable patients who have had the COVID-19 virus."* [122]

Meanwhile, the Secretary of Health Rachel Levine, removed her mother from a long-term care facility and put her in a hotel. She remained the Secretary of Health as this was uncovered and nursing home COVID-19 deaths in Pennsylvania were second highest in the country. This must be the most egregious case of insider trading ever.

Pennsylvania had a total of 4,448 patients hospitalized with COVID-19 through May 8, and 3,616 deaths. Pennsylvania has 36,022 hospital beds and 2,433 ICUs. [123]

RHODE ISLAND

Rhode Island made headlines with the first quarantine for out-of-state visitors. Drivers from New York were banned from entering Rhode Island after March 28 unless they self-quarantined or were visiting Rhode Island for work purposes. Boating was allowed, but any vessels porting in from other states were required to self-quarantine. Trout season remained open on the second Saturday in April though social distancing was required.

Rhode Island had 937 COVID-19 hospitalizations by May 8 and 399 died. Rhode Island has 2,548 hospital beds and 235 ICUs. [124]

SOUTH CAROLINA

Like most states, South Carolina limited work and travel to essential work and activities. Public beaches and parks were closed during the shutdown. Parks were under local mandates. South Carolinians protested to open South Carolina the last weekend in April. Signs like "Free South Carolina," "All businesses are essential," "End government overreach," "Freedom not fear," and "This person should be working right now," were seen as Governor Henry McMaster did allow some businesses to reopen with restrictions. McMasters said of the protests, unlike Michigan's governor Whitmer, "*This is America, come on out and say it... We might learn something.*"

South Carolina did not utilize more than 300 hospital beds and 70 ICU beds at any one time for COVID-19 patients by the peak in late April, with a capacity of 4,680 total hospital beds and 405 ICUs. Three-hundred-sixteen people died to COVID-19 by May 7, 2020.[125]

SOUTH DAKOTA

Governor Kristi Noem was a flag-bearer for light restrictions during the COVID-19 outbreak. There were no quarantines or lockdowns of South Dakota residents, though schools closed. Bars and restaurants remained open, drawing fire in the media for weeks accusing the governor of not protecting her state. Some local city mayors ordered restrictions like certain retailers to close or limit the capacity at restaurants.

Answering her critics in avoiding a stay-at-home order or mandating businesses close, Noem said, "*I just believe in our people, they know and understand personal responsibility, so I didn't mandate that any businesses closed.*" Noem did issue a stay-at-home order for vulnerable people based on the data of those who were most likely to be impacted: those with specific conditions and the elderly. She was criticized and praised for those actions largely along party lines nationally, and in the end, demonstrated what should have been done everywhere. South Dakota had 238 total COVID-19 hospitalizations and 31 deaths by May 8th, with a capacity of 153 ICUs and 4,273 total hospital beds.[126]

TEXAS

On March 22, Dallas County Judge Clay Jenkins ordered all county residents to shelter in place and nonessential businesses to close. I live in the county north adjacent to Dallas County and news of this lockdown spread like wildfire on my neighborhood's Nextdoor app that night. After months of notices on Nextdoor about urgent (!) bobcat sightings, adult complaints about kids, lost dogs and handyman referrals, the Dallas lockdown ignited discussion about our Denton County being next.

Denton County and the state of Texas were all locked down on March 24, and what Californians and New Yorkers were experiencing came home.

Non-essential businesses were closed, people flying in from New York, New Jersey, Connecticut, California, Louisiana or Washington states, or Atlanta, Chicago, Detroit and Miami were to quarantine for 14 days. With the corporate headquarters of both American Airlines and Southwest Airlines in Dallas, and DFW Airport, a major travel hub in America, this was not embraced nor followed by nearly everyone I knew still flying. It wouldn't matter as the pandemic unfolded in north Texas.

Texas is the second most populated state in America, anchored by the large cities of Houston, Dallas-Fort Worth, Austin and San Antonio. It's huge, the drive from El Paso to the Pacific Ocean takes less time than driving to Houston. It's the second largest economy in the United States, and more conservative than not, while New York and California and other "blue" states were quick to lockdown, there was some feeling among Texans that it may not follow. It would.

With knowledge about the spread and severity still a little unknown to most, and with major international airports in Dallas and Houston, would Texas experience what was happening in Detroit? A crisis like New York was never going to happen. Still, many people did catch SARS-CoV-2. Our closest family friends in north Dallas all got it, two parents in their mid-40s and two daughters aged 17 and 20. The father caught it around April 14, working at Parkland hospital in downtown Dallas, and it quickly spread within the family.

Three felt flu-like symptoms; had they not known of COVID-19, they would have assumed they caught the flu. The distinguishing impact on them was respiratory in nature, slight breathing challenges compared to the flu. Two of them lost all sense of smell and taste for about three weeks. All quarantined for about a week, felt normal and then got back out there.

A couple conscientious college students in our neighborhood wanted to help in some way, so they made care packages for healthcare workers at Parkland hospital. When they got there, they met with a nurse and said they wanted to recognize the front-line workers for all they do. The nurse laughed and said thanks but it was undeserving. Parkland was close to empty, and the nurse walked them down hallways to demonstrate how slow things were. Hallways were darkened. Rooms were empty.

Fortunately, Texas Governor Greg Abbott opened non-COVID healthcare treatments back up on April 22. Texas has 53,281 staffed hospital beds and 2,151 ICUs and three times that in ventilators. Texas would scarcely see 3,000 total hospitalized COVID-19 patients during the shutdown and 1,360 deaths by May 18.

That total increased by another thousand by the end of June. Texas loses on average 800 lives per day to all causes.

Beaumont, Texas is a small town not far from the gulf, between Houston and Louisiana. In one other law enforcement "breaking news story," Mayor Becky Ames of Beaumont "got caught" getting her nails done in a closed nail salon while donning a mask on April 21. She offered an apology and the district attorney was exploring pressing charges for her stay at home violation. Texas was not feeling effects of COVID-19 justifying the shutdowns.[127]

UTAH

Governor Gary Herbert did not issue a statewide stay-at-home order like those set by 38 other states. Herbert's directive urged Utahns to voluntarily social distance and discouraged gatherings of 10 or more people, but he did not set any penalties for people not obeying. He left it up to county officials to individually decide whether they want to back the order with the force of law. Utah did institute a two-week quarantine for those returning from out of state or exposed to a person with COVID-19 symptoms.[128]

By mid-May 2020 Utah had less than 500 total COVID-19 hospitalizations and had 61 fatalities. Utah has 5,115 total hospital beds and 482 ICU beds.[129]

WASHINGTON

Washington was an early state to act on the COVID-19 pandemic. On March 11, Governor Jay Inslee prohibited gatherings of more than 250 people in the populated King, Pierce and Snohomish counties, which does include the greater Seattle area. Schools closed as well. By March 15, bars, restaurants, fitness centers and the like closed and event limits went from 250 to 50 people. That quickly evolved to nonessential businesses limited to minimum operations or remote work, and eliminating all gatherings of people for social, spiritual and recreational purposes. State parks and recreational fisheries closed.

Washington state had a total of 2,667 hospitalized by mid-May and realized 1,016 COVID-19 deaths. Washington has 11,587 hospital beds and 1,343 ICU beds.[130]

WISCONSIN

On March 24, Governor Tony Evers ordered the closure of all nonessential businesses. Schools closed and Wisconsin mirrored Illinois's lockdown.

On April 29, while many states were opening up and some never closed in the first place, with hospitals empty and no health crisis going on in Wisconsin, The

Calumet County Sheriff's Department in Wisconsin showed up at a mother's home and reprimanded her for allowing her daughter to play at a neighbor's home for a play date. They badgered her for not strictly following the "Safer-At-Home" order. The crime was allowing two kids to play together when nothing was going on in the area, not a single child in the world was known to transmit the virus, and they'd all been locked down for more than a month.[131]

The question to ask was why the continued lockdown? Larger states had already begun to reopen their states. On May 13, the Wisconsin Supreme Court struck down the governor's order and required going forward it would require a legislative decision. It was a huge decision that would ripple to other states within days.

By mid-May, Wisconsin had 1,732 total COVID-19 hospitalizations and lost 374 lives. By now, the crisis was winding down all over the country. Wisconsin has 12,799 hospital beds and 1,180 ICU beds in the state. [132]

WYOMING

Governor Mark Gordon resisted a strict shelter-in-place order, though schools closed in March along with all other states. Most nonessential businesses closed. As a frequent visitor of Jackson Hole and the national parks, it was sad to see Grand Teton National Park and Yellowstone close, though roads in and out remained open. Camping in state parks in Wyoming closed on March 30.

Wyoming lost seven people to COVID-19 through mid-May. Wyoming has 1,953 hospital beds and 102 ICU beds in the state. When the national parks opened in late May, it was nice to see they were slammed with visitors anxious to see nature and the outdoors.

LOOKING BACK

The lockdowns would never stop the spread of COVID-19, which made the complete lockdowns such an absurd policy *with the data known*. With no cure available, cases would reappear as if they would have before the lockdowns. We locked down to prevent exceeding hospital capacity, and it was obvious by April 7 that wasn't happening anywhere.

If we look into the future into 2021, we will end where we would have anyway had the shutdowns never occurred. Countries like Japan and Sweden got it right. Fracturing the social fabric of the country, obliterating the economy was never

COVID-19: LOCKDOWNS ON TRIAL

worth it in an environment when you know the vulnerable groups were narrow and identifiable.

Preventing hospital overwhelming changed to tests and cases as debates of the lockdowns and reopening the economy began. Tests were an imperfect metric because 1) most are asymptomatic and may have or had it and would not get tested, 2) people would resist the testing if it included tracing as technology companies have proposed, 3) the testing margin of error of false negatives and false positives is below 95% reliability.[133]

Social distancing could never eliminate fatalities from COVID-19. It could delay infections and fatalities, and it probably did. After time, which we will see into 2021, we will really know what happened. When social distancing ends, COVID-19 would proceed largely as it would have without social distancing, unless many people have already developed immunity. Based on case studies discussed from Japan, Iran and some in America, that is very likely. It likely began before the lockdowns.

If you consider the lack of any hospitalizations spike over Memorial Day gatherings, including a big one at the Ozarks, as well as all of the June Black Lives Matter protests, you can see the pointlessness of any further lockdowns for COVID-19. Reporters discussed case spikes. If you ever hear anyone talking about cases without associated hospitalizations, it's worthless data.

In speaking with some doctors in Michigan about this, some argued that we prevented fatalities and therefore the lockdowns were worth it. I asked them, won't those same people then get it once we reopen and, therefore, we will be in the same situation we were in before, in total fatalities? They were silent.

To a large extent, this controversy was an exercise in data analysis with respect to the lockdowns, not medicine. With no cure in the near (2020) future, how are we doing anything but prolonging whatever the inevitable is? Second, what about the unintended fatalities of people that did not get normal course treatment of non-COVID-19 ailments?

The massive social and economic shutdowns could not stop whatever would happen, it could delay it at best. It may have to some degree, though the point is moot because hospitals never reached overcapacity. The sweeping lockdowns were the greatest domestic public policy screw up in American history.

In one of President Trump's daily COVID-19 press briefings, a reporter asked the president how many deaths were acceptable, and of course he replied "*None.*" It was such a gotcha question. You can never say "*125,000 deaths are acceptable.*" Well, you can't and get reelected. But it's an impossible standard those perpetuating the lockdowns would endure.

It's also a standard none of us live by. If none were acceptable, literally none, then no one would drive, fly, climb a ladder, my son and I for sure would not be climbing mountains. No one would smoke, drink, boat, the list is endless, isn't it? Three million people die every year in America, 8,000 Americans lose their life every day. Cancer claims the most, at 20%. And any given year the flu claims 50,000. Around 40,000 people die each year from car accidents. I lost a close friend in his 40s a decade ago to pancreatic cancer, and it sucks when someone leaves us prematurely. I lost a cousin to COVID-19 in a care facility in Detroit.

The early data showed us that this was going to be a painful time for many people, but not for most people. The data told us that a month before the lockdowns. At some point you make the hard decision to carry on and protect those most vulnerable. Had we done that, it's probable at the end of 2020 we would end where we would have had no state ever locked down.

In an analysis published on May 11 by the Dornsife School of Public Health at Drexel University, they concluded that the stay-at-home order saved 232,878 lives.[134] The article was based on a model in *The New York Times* from March 25, which means the model inputs had to be a combination of either the Imperial College or the IHME, both of which at that date were grossly overstated. This analysis was pushed out by *The Hill*. Data analysis continued using bad assumptions for longer than we would have expected by May.

CHAPTER 10

THE CARES ACT

On February 12, just over one month after the CDC announced a detection of COVID-19, the Dow hit an all-time high, well over 29,000.[135] A month and a half later, on March 27, President Trump was signing the Coronavirus Aid, Relief, and Economic Security Act, shortened as the "CARES" Act. The $2 trillion economic stimulus package was created to offset a 30% fall in the DJIA and impending tens of millions unemployed, and companies on the brink of bankruptcy.

Two days before, when the Senate first approved the bill 96-0, the U.S. coronavirus death toll was nearing 1,000.[136] The "CARES" Act sought to provide aid in a variety of ways to businesses, hospitals, and individuals. Let's take a look at some of the impactful and noteworthy parts of the bill. Below are some highlights. One could write a book just about the CARES Act and a critique, but that's beyond the scope of this book. Our scope is more around actions that would have never required a CARES Act in the first place.

UNEMPLOYMENT BENEFITS

By the time the CARES Act was passed, jobless claims dwarfed the 210,000 average weekly new claims. How many millions of new claims was speculative, but that number reached 40 million before we turned the corner. Around 40 million jobs were lost in a couple of weeks. Forty million.

The CARES Act provided jobless workers an additional $600 per week for four months, concluding at the end of July.[137] This is stacked on top of state unemployment benefits, which is lower than $600/month in 40 U.S. states.[138] Furthermore, the bill includes unemployment benefits to those who are jobless because of the virus but do not qualify for regular benefits (e.g. the self-employed, independent contractors, etc.). Additionally, there is a 13-week extension on the state benefits, which normally last 26 weeks, in most states. Unemployment benefits total $260 billion.

Below are some of the highest and lowest unemployment benefits by state.[139] As mentioned above, in 40 of 50 states, the weekly benefit is less than $600.

Highest:

- Massachusetts – $1,220 (variable range)
- Ohio – $802
- Washington – $790
- Rhode Island – $730
- Connecticut – $724

Lowest:

- Mississippi – $235
- Arizona – $240
- Louisiana – $247
- Alabama – $275
- Florida – $275

Senator Lindsey Graham led the rationale of the blanketed $600 stacking of federal benefits. If the average state's weekly unemployment benefits was approximately $475, and unemployment individuals can receive up to $600 from the federal government until the end of July, that is the equivalent of earning an income above a rate of $50,000 annually for a third of 2020.

This figure is more than many people make annually (the real median personal income in the U.S. is just under $34,000, which would equate to a little over $11,000 per third of the year).[140] Before some analysis, a quick comment that for all the money state and federal governments take and spend, anything going back to taxpayers is great.

Graham said that, "*this bill pays you more not to work than if you were working,*" and this group of legislators claimed that the temporarily expanded funds would disincentivize people from keeping jobs or returning to work.[141] If the economy was to reopen prior to the end of July, many businesses, and therefore the economy, would be hurt because it would be more beneficial to many individuals to stay home and continue collecting unemployment checks.

July was right around the corner. If the federal government could give rich universities millions of dollars they don't need, we can consider the extra unemployment payment "pain and suffering" compensation for those who lost their jobs due to the government action around COVID-19.

My belief is that most people would rather work than collect unemployment if they could, particularly knowing it had an expiration. Whatever disincentive there was to return to work would eventually pass.

INDIVIDUAL DIRECT PAYMENTS

Per the U.S. Department of the Treasury:

> "The CARES Act provides for Economic Impact Payments to American households of up to $1,200 per adult for individuals whose income was less than $99,000 (or $198,000 for joint filers) and $500 per child under 17 years old – or up to $3,400 for a family of four.
>
> Additionally, the IRS will use the information on the Form SSA-1099 and Form RRB-1099 to generate $1,200 Economic Impact Payments to Social Security recipients who did not file tax returns in 2018 or 2019. Recipients will receive these payments as a direct deposit or by paper check, just as they would normally receive their benefits."[142]

These direct payments to eligible taxpayers total approximately $290 billion. Question: why would the government pay individuals money if their employment was not interrupted?

While direct stimulus payments to individuals can be a sort of non-labor income that disincentivizes working, it has been seen that these types of payments have been helpful in times of recession. Claudia Sahm,[143] who formerly served on the Board of Governors of the Federal Reserve, wrote a chapter in an academic work on fiscal policy in times of recession. While *the effectiveness of stimulus payments in a recession largely depends on the spending response of households...empirical evidence. . . across numerous research studies of the Great Recession [of 2008-2009] strongly suggests that at least some forms of stimulus to households can measurably boost spending in the near term.*[144]

When demand and consumption increase in times of recession or economic uncertainty, the job market strengthens and prices find a healthy (or at least healthier) equilibrium.

STUDENTS

While college students received no direct money from the government (yet their universities did and were enabled to distribute aid to students in need), the bill provides a suspension on all federal loans until September 30. In other words, there are no required payments on loans owned by the Department of Education through the end of the third quarter. Question: Why would this be blanketed for all student loans, rather than those associated with students/graduates that suffered an employment setback? Regardless, it was short term relief and it too would pass.

HOSPITALS

Hospitals and healthcare providers received approximately $100 billion as a result of the bill (this money goes toward the Public Health and Social Services Emergency Fund).[145] These funds went toward reimbursements for COVID-19 care and lost revenue – buying supplies, training new HC workers, hiring new employees, increasing capacity. Considering the government basically bankrupted the healthcare system during a healthcare crisis, this one was obvious.

As covered in other chapters, nearly all hospitals were going broke because of the lockdowns. With no non-emergency and non-COVID-19 activity, and with no COVID-19 activity in most hospitals, hospital revenue fell substantially. For example, the UCSD Health Center (San Diego), by April 28, had "lost more than $50 million in revenue since March."[146] Small private practices were hit harder than hospitals mostly because they would not have the reserves as patient visits fell drastically. This reality drove thousands of healthcare layoffs.

The hospital and private practice payments of the CARES Act and other bills helped with employee retention, but most of the money was directed toward COVID-19 care and, in the case of lost revenue, was not nearly enough to make up the deficit. In the end, what an irony that the healthcare industry was hemorrhaging money during a healthcare pandemic.

AIRLINE INDUSTRY

The CARES Act outlines human services pandemic relief for the air industry:

> "Notwithstanding any other provision of law, to preserve aviation jobs and compensate air carrier industry workers, the Secretary shall provide financial assistance that shall exclusively be used for the continuation of payment of employee wages, salaries, and benefits to—
>
> (1) passenger air carriers, in an aggregate amount up to $25,000,000,000;
>
> (2) cargo air carriers, in the aggregate amount up to $4,000,000,000; and
>
> (3) contractors, in an aggregate amount up to $3,000,000,000."[147]

Any of the airlines receiving benefits were to retain 90% of their employees through September 2020. Great call. Any executives at a benefiting airline must also have a ceiling of $3MM in annual compensation, and no one making more than $425,000 would be able to get a raise until a year after the loan is repaid. The government certainly caused this crisis, but you could make a good argument that executive compensation should have been limited to far less than $3MM and those making more than $200,000 a year be subject to a temporary pay decrease.

EDUCATION

Thirty billion dollars was provisioned for local school systems and higher education. Depending on the size of the state, each governor was allotted $3B, half of which was to go directly to students for aid. Half of all funds were to go to colleges and universities. Some news was made when some very well-off colleges, like Harvard, were given grants and still laid off support staff when students left campus. Given no students were refunded any tuition for the spring semester and actual costs of operations on campuses had to go down, you have to wonder why the schools needed or received so much money.

Harvard, Stanford, Penn, Yale and others ended up declining their grants given they have so few low-income students to whom they would provide relief, as well as their large endowments.

On May 6, the Department of Education required any institutions receiving aid provide an easy to understand reconciliation of where exactly the funds went on their websites. Great call. Still, with many schools having billion-dollar endowments, why? Where did their cost structure increase?

OTHER GRANTS

Some other puzzling things were included in the CARES Act. Not sure how these are directly related to the pandemic, you be the judge:

- $1B to recapitalize Amtrack: perhaps because they are in tough financial shape anyway and they would suffer lost revenues with everyone locked down
- $10B in grants for airports, perhaps also making up for lost revenues
- $400MM in election assistance for states. Why would this be included in a March 2020 bill? If necessary, why not wait a few months as we neared the election to determine where we would be?

SMALL BUSINESSES

Between money allocated for small business administration loans, salaries, expenses, entrepreneurial programs, and other related entities or initiatives, there is approximately $377 billion in new grants and loans for small businesses.[148]

LARGER CORPORATIONS

There was an expansion of $500 billion for lending to businesses and local governments.[149] In the four weeks since the first stimulus bill, approximately 22 million Americans filed unemployment claims and most businesses were closed.[150] On Friday, April 24, President Trump signed a second stimulus package into law. This next piece of relief legislation, totaling $484 billion, was directed at small businesses and hospitals. The relief can be broken down as follows:

- $310 billion → Paycheck Protection Program (PPP), which mainly helps businesses with under 500 employees, small lenders and banks, and mid-sized credit unions and banks
- $60 billion → Economic Injury Disaster Loan program, "which reaches communities and small businesses in underserved areas"
- $75 billion → hospitals
- $25 billion → expand virus testing[151]

So, what did the people have to say?

REACTIONS TO THE CARES ACT

Speaker of the House Nancy Pelosi (D-CA) called the bill a "mitigation" of COVID-19's destruction and foresaw the government pursuing more recovery efforts down the road.[152] In the upper chamber, Senate Majority Leader Mitch McConnell said that the CARES Act would "help the people of this country weather this storm."[153]

In the White House, President Trump signed the bill and said that it would *"deliver urgently needed relief,"* thanking both parties for putting Americans first (after endless debate between party leaders that almost resulted in no stimulus bill at all).[154] McConnell joined Trump at the White House, saying it was a *"proud moment for our country."*[155]

In New York, which experienced approximately 70% of the coronavirus-related deaths in the U.S. at the time, Governor Andrew Cuomo called the bill "irresponsible" and "reckless." Cuomo claimed that the bill did not meet needs for New York, which was set to receive approximately $5 billion, and expressed his disappointment.[156]

Ben Shapiro, a conservative opinion writer, after reflecting on the unnecessary *"pork"* in the bill (such as millions of dollars to the Kennedy Center), said it *"on any normal level... is a bunch of crap."* However, he supported the bill in that it appeared that the options were *"a pork-laden bleep show or nothing, and this is going to allow businesses to continue to operate for the next three months, [so] okay."*[157]

Bill Maher, another popular political commentator, has been a vocal critic of President Trump and supported Bernie Sanders and then Hillary Clinton in the

2016 election cycle. In late April, he interviewed Nancy Pelosi about the bill and questioned her clear support for the multiple bills passed. He asked her,

> *"That's a lot of money, you know, in a very short period of time. I know Congress controls the purse strings. I can't imagine there's much left in the purse. I just don't get it. I don't understand how – I know we can bailout certain sectors, as we have done in the past. I don't know how you can just keep indefinitely writing checks. We were $20 trillion in the hole to begin with. And all world governments, who are already in debt, are doing this. How can the whole world be writing this funny money?"*

And after Speaker Pelosi discussed the unique life-and-death nature of the public health crisis, he responded,

> *"Well, [the economy] will recover unless people get wise to the fact we're just writing checks for money that doesn't exist. I mean – what is the point of bailing out banks who are just going to loan back the money that doesn't exist to us again? It seems like it's a house of cards that could, in the end, wind up hurting more people than the disease."*[158]

Mark Cuban, owner of our nearby Dallas Mavericks basketball team and known for his work on the show, Shark Tank, has often been a vocal critic of the President. However, he became a supporter for at least the end of March, quickly expressing support for the bill. Sounding like a teenager, he called it *"literally the best stimulus bill ever for small businesses."* He went on to connect it to his first company and said small businesses need to know about the PPP (mentioned above). He even provided a call to action: *"So, if you are an entrepreneur, if you're a small business operator, you need to be cognizant and you need to apply ASAP."*[159] Cuban also showed respect for President Trump stepping aside for experts, saying, *"I give him all the credit in the world."*[160]

MONETARY POLICY AT THE FED: INTEREST RATES AND BONDS

On Sunday, March 15, the Fed "cut interest rates to essentially zero on Sunday and launched a massive $700 billion quantitative easing program to shelter the economy from the effects of the virus."[161] Quantitative easing (QE) is an unconventional monetary policy in which the Fed purchases longer-term bonds. These bonds are usually government bonds but not always. Put simply:

QE → increase in longer-term prices → decrease in government interest rates (longer-term) → decrease in corporate interest rates (longer-term)

Lower interest rates allow for increased investment, of course. The use of the unconventional QE is beneficial, to use one example, in the world of oil. In mid-to-late April, there was a shocking oil price crisis: "Ongoing concerns over swelling oil inventories, with little demand to ease the pile up due to the ongoing fallout from the coronavirus, sent West Texas Intermediate crude for May delivery plunging 305 percent to a record low -$36.73 per barrel. At a price below zero, buyers were paid to take delivery as there are costs associated with transportation and storage."[162] Relatively quickly, the prices had come back above the surface.[163] So, what does QE have to do with oil prices?

Many U.S. investment banks have money in U.S. oil companies. If the latter go bankrupt, it is possible that the banks follow suit. The Fed responding with QE, by purchasing corporate bonds in this case, seeks to keep these companies and banks afloat. When they purchase these bonds, the companies receive money from the Fed.

CHAPTER 11

DESOLATION BOULEVARD

Over the last few years, my son and I took up mountain climbing. We enjoyed the planning, the training, the connection under pressure. We had some great adventures and were able to get deep into our national parks in the Tetons, Yosemite and many climbs in Colorado. In 2018, a movie came out that won an Academy Award for best documentary. We were very excited to see *Free Solo*, a documentary of Alex Honnold's climb up El Capitan's 3,000-foot vertical face by himself with no protection (rope). It's the greatest athletic achievement in history. If you doubt that, spend some time climbing in the mountains and let's regroup.

In watching dozens of interviews with Honnold about what happened during his climb, the inevitable questions he is always asked are "Were you afraid of dying?" "Why take the risk?" and "Why do this if one little slip will be unrecoverable?" His answer is always about balancing risk and consequence.

Honnold isn't a reckless daredevil. He's a very deep thinker and is very analytical. His response to those questions is always that while the consequence (of falling) is great, he feels the risk is low due to his preparation and understanding of the circumstances.

The leaders of America, from President Trump to each governor, would have to make enormous risk and consequence calculations. What are the consequences of shutting down the economy and society, and what is the health risk if we don't? Most leaders, in America and around the world, bet that the health risk was too great and worth the consequential economic and social crashes.

The problem is that they misunderstood the risk in a way that Honnold understood his level of risk. Our health risk was much less than anyone outside Japan and Sweden thought, and the consequences of those decisions impacted hundreds of millions of people as the economy fell off the cliff.

Starting off 2020, the U.S. economy was performing at its highest level in decades. Unemployment was the lowest in 50 years, and at a historical record low for women, blacks, whites, Hispanics, youth, every segment you care pull out. Even into the second week of March 2020, the data was strong. New job postings were up.

By the second week of March, it was like sitting on a Florida beach enjoying calm winds and low waves rolling in but seeing on The Weather Channel the growing disturbance of a tropical storm brewing in the east Atlantic miles away. Within days, that tropical storm would grow to a Category 5 hurricane dwarfing Hurricanes Andrew or Michael as it made landfall.

MARKET IMPLICATIONS

The stock market reacted to the imminent landfall before the layoffs and closures began. At the end of February, the major market indexes shed 20% in value mostly based on the shutdowns in China disrupting supply chains and their consumption of goods alone. The first week of March saw a bump back of about 10%, and the following three weeks saw a gradual decline of 40% before bouncing back up when the CARES Act was passed.

When President Trump would tout the stock market growth as one of his performance scorecards, critics would often counter that it's limiting because so many millions of people are not investors and shareholders. Only 55% of Americans are invested in the stock market. The stock market declines would have impacts that would far extend from individual investors.

For example, public pensions are heavily invested in the stock market. These represent retirements for teachers, firefighters and city employees. If pension costs go up, or there isn't enough money to fund them from investment declines, one of two things have to happen. They have to get more funding, which either means higher taxes or borrowing. Or, they have to reduce their costs in other areas, which can mean a decrease in other local services or layoffs to save on expenses. This is a big reason it's difficult for teachers to get raises.[164] It's not unlike challenges the U.S. automakers faced. Union healthcare costs and pensions made domestic cars more expense than comparable foreign cars. That's not a criticism of unions at all, they serve a great role for our workers, it's just an economic fact.

HURRICANE UNEMPLOYMENT

On March 11, 2020, President Trump ceased all travel to most countries, and by the time California locked down on March 20, businesses had already done so all over the country. In just that time frame, hundreds of employers began shedding their employees with no revenues to support them:

- Marriott began furloughing tens of thousands of employees
- McMenamins, an Oregon restaurant group, began laying off 3,000 employees
- Ports around the country were laying off drivers since supply chains were largely compromised and their customers were compressing their businesses
- Hotels and casinos were laying off thousands of employees
- Thousands of restaurants across the country closed their doors, hoping to open up when this passed but as we saw, many would not
- Malls all over the country were closing and major retailers immediately furloughed employees
- Air Canada laid off 5,000 flight attendants
- The Cheesecake Factory had 294 locations and 38,000 employees. Almost immediately TCF closed 27 restaurants and informed their landlords they would not be able to meet April 1 rent, and that's with two weeks of shutdown
- Theme parks like Sea World and Disney furloughed nearly all their park employees

In March alone, 10 million people filed initial unemployment claims. Ten million people. That after a weekly average of about 210,000 for the past year. The new claims during the height of the lockdowns are over the page.

The unemployment claims reached 30 million people by the end of April and 40 million in May. Forty million people. The layoffs were further-reaching than in March:

- Honda and Nissan each laid off 10,000 employees. General Motors and other automakers combined for tens of thousands of layoffs
- Qwest Diagnostics laid off 4,000 people. Think about that: in a healthcare pandemic the foremost healthcare testing organization was getting crushed. Qwest earns a large share of their revenues from new and existing employee testing. With no new employees and a shrinking workforce, they were left dry. Still, a healthcare testing business and one of the largest private organizations able to do coronavirus testing on the survival edge in a pandemic?

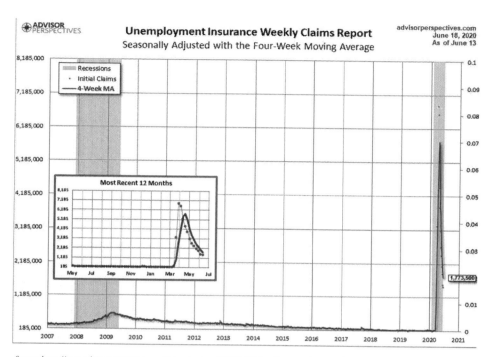

Source: https://www.advisorperspectives.com/dshort/updates/2020/06/18/weekly-unemployment-claims-1-51m-down-58k-from-last-week

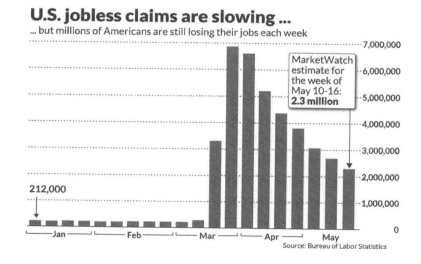

Source: https://www.marketwatch.com/story/jobless-claims-since-pandemic-set-to-hit-39-million-but-the-more-important-number-to-watch-is-how-many-are-collecting-benefits-2020-05-20

144

- Under Armour, Dick's Sporting Goods, Best Buy, L Brands, The Gap, Macy's JC Penney, Kohl's, practically every major brick and mortar retailer, a couple million employees combined.
- In all, a population equivalent to the state of Texas, the second largest state in the union, would lose their jobs within three weeks

INDUSTRIES MOST AFFECTED

RETAIL
This one should be obvious. With everything non-essential closed for two months in most places in a best-case scenario, the retail industry was crushed. The advent of online shopping had already ruptured malls and many retailers. COVID-19 would quite possibly be the end to iconic brands like JC Penney and Neiman Marcus. Penney's filed for bankruptcy in May. Millions of retail employees would be laid off or furloughed.

Apparel retailer sales were cut in half year-over-year for March, and in April, more than 75% down. Furniture stores, eat-in food retailers, gas stations, bookstores, all would be down to next to nothing year-over-year by May 1. The retail industry employs one in 10 working people in the country. Only the healthcare industry makes up a higher percentage of American workers.

The National Restaurant Association estimated the restaurant industry lost $25 billion in sales and 3 million jobs just in March, with the sales number likely doubled through April.

TRAVEL
This one is obvious too. The federal government allocated billions for the airline industry in the CARES Act amidst the shutdown. The International Air Transport Association estimates the airline industry would lose $314 billion in revenues in 2020, worse than any worst case ever modeled for them. The recipients were American Airlines, Delta Airlines, Southwest Airlines, JetBlue and United Airlines. Thirty percent of those grants would have to be repaid and in some cases the government may take stock ownership of them.

Airlines in the United States employ 750,000 people. Major layoffs were avoided early in the pandemic, but flight travel was down 95%. TSA estimated they screened 2,000,000 passengers a day in America in April 2019, and that dropped to 100,000 per day in April 2020. With businesses and vacation travel nearly halted, no one was flying.

For the airline industry to pick up, businesses needed to resume travel for their employees. Still, it's unlikely the industry would see any material recovery in 2020. Flights moved to open middle seats and masks required. For air travelers, that may be a decent tradeoff as seat and leg space had been reduced in recent years.

The hotel industry was completely decimated by the shutdowns. Compare these charts of how much more the COVID-19 shutdowns have hurt the hotel industry compared to past recessions.[165]

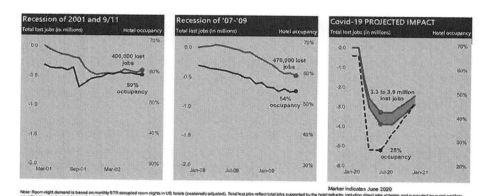

Note: Room night demand is based on monthly STR occupied room nights in US hotels (seasonally adjusted). Total lost jobs reflect total jobs supported by the hotel industry, including direct jobs at hotels and supported by guest ancillary spending (e.g., restaurants), as well as indirect (supply-chain) jobs, and induced jobs supported by wages and salaries of direct employees.
Source: STR, BEA, BLS, Oxford Economics

Source: https://www.hotelmanagement.net/own/studies-break-down-covid-19-s-impact-hotels-travel-plans

Occupancy rates dropped down to 10%, which means nearly all hotel rooms were empty each day. Convention hotels would likely remain vacant well into at least the Fall of 2020. The interesting thing about the travel impact is that even though the virus would prove to be more harmful than the flu only to a specific and now-identified segment of the population, the fear of it would linger on. Even with so many people testing positive and not getting seriously ill, from celebrities to media figures to athletes, the media was not doing a good job of offering balance and positive information about COVID-19. As long as fear was prevailing, hotels would have no chance of recovering.

OIL AND GAS

Crude oil prices dropped in April to a 50-year low. The combination of new technology to produce it and new reserves discovered drove the price of oil down in the late 2010's. The world produces about 80 million barrels of oil per day. It's hard to fathom how much the earth has at that level of production. The United States became the world's largest oil producer of late, producing 15 million barrels a day to Saudi Arabia's 12 million barrels per day.

Two factors led to the oil and gas industry's near-collapse in 2020. Russia, not a member of OPEC, and Saudi Arabia entered into a price war because Russia refused to drop oil production as consumption started to drop when the pandemic began. Saudi Arabia sought to reduce production to keep prices stable. As that happened, consumption dropped like we've never seen. Jet fuel consumption fell almost 75% in April, and gasoline consumption dropped in half year-over-year, both worldwide.

On several cable news reports in April, some analysts and politicians scoffed at the oil industry and made some light comments about how great it is gas prices are dropping, almost placing the oil and gas industry a notch above pornography. However, the oil and gas industry is the foundation of much of our economy. The oil and natural gas industry in America supports 10.3 million jobs and nearly 8 percent of our GDP, and more than a trillion dollars to our economy. If the oil and gas industry collapses, so do we.

The list is almost endless of industries affected and the commensurate number of people they employ who would lose their jobs. Why does it matter? Because with less or no income, they spend less, thus making them unable to support other industries, like hospitality, food and beverage, or retail. It's all interconnected and would have far-reaching impacts in all industries.

MILK AND CHEESE

With schools, restaurants and coffee shops closed, the food industry became decimated like other industries. With a sharp decline in consumption, milk prices dropped and products like milk and cheese, which have a shelf life, would end up going to waste. Dairy cows are milked two to three times a day, and that milk has to get processed within 72 hours. If there is no end user to consume it, it's wasted. The industry received a bailout, but in a low-margin industry without deep reserves, the farming community was getting crushed.

SMALL BUSINESSES

Small businesses were hit hardest from the lockdowns. A small business is defined as having 500 or fewer employees. There are more than 30 million small businesses in America, and they comprise more than 99% of all businesses. Small businesses employ nearly 60 million people, almost half of the workforce. Around 45% of the United States' GDP is generated from small businesses.

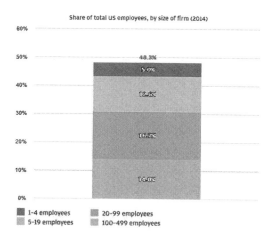

Share of total US employees, by size of firm (2014)

Nearly half of all people who work are employed by small businesses.

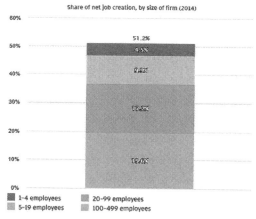

Share of net job creation, by size of firm (2014)

Small businesses account for more than half of all jobs created in the United States.

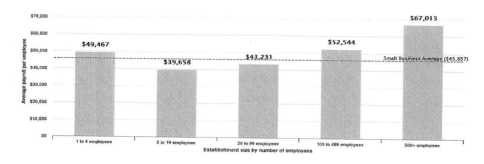

Small businesses are classified in sub-segments. Many are non-employer businesses where no employees are present except the owner, like a real estate agent, someone providing services like an attorney practicing alone, a personal coach, or a sole proprietor trades person like a plumber or electrician. Next are employer small businesses, like restaurants, a personal care salon, small manufacturers and fabricators.

Finally, there are high-growth small businesses, such as in high-technology manufacturing and services. Non-employer small businesses make up three quarters of all small businesses. According to JP Morgan Chase, non-employer small businesses have a little more than 60 days of cash reserves, on average, and employer small businesses have half that.

Wallethub conducted several interesting surveys at the end of April. In one survey, 87% of small business owners said they "were hurting over the shutdowns" and 35% said they could only last a total of three months before going out of business. One-third had laid off employees and another third intended to lay off employees.[166]

HEALTHCARE INDUSTRY

At a first glance, one would have expected in a healthcare pandemic that the healthcare industry would be busy and experiencing record revenues. In the greatest irony of the shutdown period, the healthcare industry was suffering as much as any of the major industries.

Governors directed primary care physicians to stop seeing patients for fear of a spread of the virus. The things that keep family practitioners in business, like routine physicals, diagnosing and prescribing for typical ailments, and facilitating lab work practically evaporated overnight. Family practitioners are usually single physician to a handful of physicians per office, with 3-4 office and nurse staff per doctor.

On April 5, I called my primary care physician's office to have them place a prescription refill. I've been going there for a decade and have no health issues. I'd just had a full physical with lab work on February 6. The nurse there said I was required to have a "tele-visit" with my doctor in order for them to call the refill in. I complained about having to do this (and be charged) having just been there. At this point, my prescription was held hostage and spring allergies were getting bad.

My doctor shared this with me: their office had four doctors and saw on average 70 patients per day. The doctor's office was unable to see patients and they'd laid off half their staff. Their only way to make money to stay afloat was to charge for tele-visits ($52 for me) for prescription refills. If things did not open soon, they would shut down.

He went on to say that doctors on staff at Baylor-Scott, a major hospital organization in Texas, would keep their doctors on the payroll until June but if things did not pick up, they'd be letting them go. I was shocked. I called my surgeon brother in Michigan and he confirmed. Healthcare providers were going broke in the midst of a healthcare crisis.

What may have been 70 patient visits in a day moved to 13 tele-visits with a much lower charge (revenue for them). You may be thinking doctors are all wealthy and can afford anything, or that they are all high-income earners, but they are also small business owners. They support a staff, pay rent, many have student loans, it's also a high-cost structure. As soon as they are unable to see patients, it would not take long before they have to close the doors.

If patients could not tele-visit, either not figuring out how to use Zoom or tele-conference, they were often left out. Insurance companies have certain requirements for a tele-visit. Suppose many of the tele-visits were not just prescription refills like mine. Diagnosing a new illness over the phone would not be easy. If a patient was ill, they would need to go to an urgent care facility or a hospital. That means, if they have insurance, higher copays, and if no insurance, a much higher cost.

The CARES Act helped subsidize these doctors for a couple months if they did not lay off any employees. Fortunately, it would not last even a couple months in many states, as many began reopening in early May. It's likely their volume would go down because so many patients would lose their jobs and insurance or be afraid to go to the doctor for fear of catching the virus.

Specialists also saw decreases in business. Urologists, obstetricians, orthopedics, they all experienced severe reductions in work. Many small private practices had been bought out by hospitals in recent years, turning small-business-owner physicians into hospital employees. The pandemic shutdowns would threaten existing private practices even more. Dentists? Their offices closed for at least a couple of months. .

In the state-by-state reviews, we compared actual COVID-19 hospitalizations to hospital capacity. With no ability to perform non-emergency services and waiting for a flood of COVID-19 patients that never materialized, hospitals were hemorrhaging money, pushing them to the brink.

Beaumont Health is Michigan's largest hospital network with eight hospitals in the metro Detroit area. Beaumont laid off 2,475 of its 38,000 employees and eliminated 450 jobs as their revenue dropped in April 2020. Eighty-five to 90% of their surgical procedures fell off during the COVID-19 flurry. The highest number of COVID-19 patients the Beaumont system saw in hard-hit Detroit on their peak day was 1,274 on April 10. Beaumont has nearly 18,000 hospital beds in total.

Hospitals began seeing drops in revenue of up to 70%. Small town hospitals with no cases or COVID-19 hospitalizations furloughed employees, laid them off and outright closed during the lockdowns. Almost half of all small-town hospitals were losing money before the pandemic hit, and without the ability to perform non-emergencies, they would fracture even more.[167]

Many second-tier hospitals and those in smaller communities may only have sixty days of cash reserves on hand to weather the downturn. Even before the lockdowns, 125 small-town hospitals closed in the last 10 years and another nearly 500 are close to closing. This would make healthcare even more precious to those in need outside larger cities.[168]

PRIVATE HOSPITAL ORGANIZATIONS[169]

Large hospital organizations have deeper reserves than small practices, but they were crushed just the same. Below are some of the largest hospital groups in the country:

HCA Healthcare, based in Nashville, TN employs 38,000 physicians and 94,000 registered nurses, and they receive more than 30 million patients a year, nearly nine million emergency room visits.

Ascension Health based in St. Louis, MS, is the second largest hospital group with 151 hospitals. Others with more than a hundred hospitals in its domain include CommonSpirit Heath from Chicago, Community Health Systems also in Tennessee (Like HCA).

Trinity Health (Livonia, MI.): 92 hospitals. Trinity Health is a Catholic health system with 92 hospitals and 107 continuing care locations. It employs around 129,000 individuals, including 7,800 physicians and clinicians. The health system has locations in 22 states and serves communities that include about 30 million people nationwide.

LifePoint Health (Brentwood, TN.): 86 hospitals. The National Rural Health Association recognized two of the health system's hospitals — Riverview Regional Medical Center in Carthage, TN, and Trousdale Medical Center in Hartsville, TN — among the top 20 critical-access hospitals in the nation.

Tenet Healthcare and Baylor Scott and White Health are both based in Dallas and respectively have 65 and 48 hospitals. Tenet has 65 acute-care hospitals and 475 outpatient centers and serves 10 million patients a year, employing 110,000 people. Tenet furloughed an undisclosed number of employees in the Spring of 2020.

Baylor Scott has 800 care sites and 7,800 physicians on staff. Kaiser Permanente based in Oakland California has 39 hospitals, 697 medical offices and employs

23,000 physicians-- more than 200,000 people overall. These are just some of the very large providers of healthcare that employ millions of people across all large hospital networks.

The American Hospital Association ballparked that collectively hospitals were losing up to $50 billion in April alone. They had a decrease in non-emergency procedures, an increase in COVID-19-related expenses (personal protective equipment, training), and an increase in uninsured patients coming in for emergencies because normal care facilities like doctor's offices were closed.

1.4MM health-care jobs disappeared in April 2020, which included nearly 135,000 hospital jobs, 243,000 at physician offices and more than 500,000 at dental offices. The healthcare sector represented 7% of all April job losses. [170]

Even as they reopened in May, in most states, the flow of patients was slow to ramp up because not all patients seeking non-emergency care were comfortable going in. *The Washington Post* reported that Michigan's Beaumont hospital group went from earning about $16 million each month to losing about $100 million a month in April.[171] Bon Secours Mercy Health based in Cincinnati has 48 hospitals and employs more than 60,000 people, and it reported having lost $100 million in April.

While the data early on from the cruise ships and in analyzing who was getting sick, needing ventilators and dying in other countries like Italy (their wave hit before America's) never indicated hospitals would globally be at or over capacity, all hospitals were forced to put all their chips in for COVID-19 and lost big on that. The CARES Act gave hospitals huge bailouts, at a cost to taxpayers. With the debt so high already, it's hard to know how or when that debt will ever catch up.

PHARMACEUTICALS

For one other validation that people with non-COVID-19 illnesses were staying away from healthcare, consider this. Merck is a $46B pharmaceuticals company, making therapeutic and preventive drug agents and vaccines, as well as animal health products, most by prescription. Merck communicated to investors they expect prescription drug sales will drop by $1.7 billion year-over-year because many patients (customers) were staying away from their doctors. Animal health drugs were forecasted to drop $400 million.

Patients with chronic conditions were not receiving normal care and that would have an unintended consequence on those people as COVID-19 monopolized healthcare in 2020, all with hospitals going empty and doctors' offices going broke.[172]

Johnson and Johnson is a $80B company that makes everything from medical devices to over the counter healthcare products to pharmaceuticals. With elective and preventive procedures down, Johnson and Johnson saw a drop in revenues and dropped their 2Q and 2020 revenue forecast. Below is how the pandemic and a loss in revenues affected the stocks of the following pharmaceutical companies.

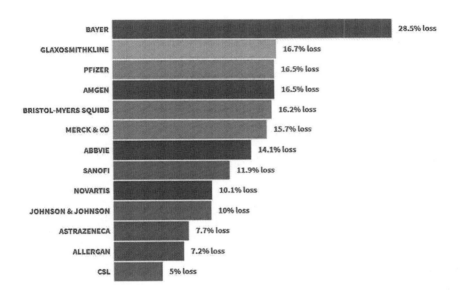

Source: https://www.fiercepharma.com/pharma/covid-19-drained-2-6-trillion-market-value-from-big-pharma-q1-but-gilead-and-regeneron

OPPORTUNITY COST

In the United Kingdom, cancer kills 450 people a day, more than 160,000 people a year. A group of UK oncologists estimated that 60,000 more cancer patients could die because of a lack of treatment or diagnosis. In an average April, oncologists would see 30,000 cancer patients in the UK, and in April 2020, that dropped to about 5,000.[173]

The American Cancer Society reported on a Survivor Views survey in April 2020. In that survey, patients responded on the impact the COVID-19 monopolization of healthcare resources would have on them:

- *Half (51%) of all those surveyed reported some impact on their care due to the virus. Of those who've experienced an effect, nearly 1 in 4 report a delay in care or treatment. Among those 1 in 4, the most common delays were for in-person provider appointments (50%); delayed access to imaging services to determine if a patient's cancer had grown or returned (20%); access to supportive services, including physical therapy or mental health care (20%); and access to surgical procedures (8%).*

- *Among just the respondents who remain in active treatment, more than a quarter (27%) report a delay in their care, and 13% say they don't know when it will be rescheduled.*
- *Cancer patients are also feeling economic stress in the wake of the pandemic. Nearly 4 in 10 (38%) respondents say COVID-19 is having a notable effect on their ability to afford their care, due mostly to reduced work hours (14%).*
- *Reduced work hours and lost jobs are of particular concern because these have the potential to impact access to health insurance. Of the respondents who reported that they or a family member living with them had lost a job, 43% had employer-sponsored coverage. Of those who reported they or a family member had their hours reduced, 58% percent had employer-sponsored health insurance.*
- *Nearly half of those earning $30,000 or less say they're worried about affording their care (46%); more than a third (34%) of those earning up to $60,000 are worried and a quarter (25%) of those earning up to $110,000 are concerned.[174]*

On May 6 2020, the Stop TB Partnership published a whitepaper on the effects the lockdowns would have worldwide on the spread of tuberculosis.[175] They estimated the increase in TB could grow to more than a million incremental cases because of the lockdowns worldwide. The study focused on India, Kenya and Ukraine. The studies from these countries was then extrapolated to the rest of the world. TB is the biggest infectious disease killer worldwide. Around 1.5 million people die from it every year. The mortality rate from TB infection is about 3%, significantly higher than COVID-19.

Below is their projection of increased TB incidence and deaths. The baseline is what is expected, the red line represents a two-month lockdown and two-month restoration, which is likely to be the case. In that scenario, they estimate 342,000 incremental deaths. On the date of this publication, less than 300,000 COVID-19 deaths had been reported worldwide and far less all-cause mortality increases worldwide.

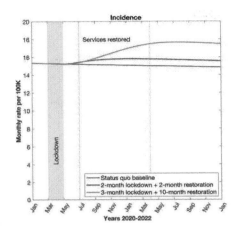
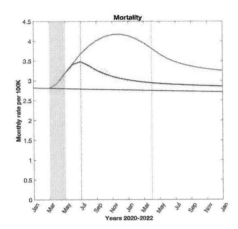

Many doctors and hospital administrators with whom I spoke in researching this book said they would be playing catch-up with treatments for non-COVID-19 patients. One said he expected an "apocalyptic" surge in treatments and even fatalities from those who did not receive normal cycles of treatments. If that happens, is it a layered effect?

If there is a number of increased non-COVID-19 deaths due to the lack of healthcare that was preempted by preparation for a COVID-19 healthcare surge that never happened, are those COVID-19 deaths too? Or, should they reduce the net COVID-19 death impact because from an all-cause mortality point of view, those deaths would not have occurred, thus displacing COVID-19 death totals? The sweeping impact of COVID-19 on the healthcare system would be the most colossal misappropriation of resources in American history.

Below is an evaluation of consumer healthcare spending in April 2020 compared to April 2019. In much of the country including the more populated urban areas, hospital spending was down more than 50% year-over-year.

Into June, it's estimated that more than 90 million Americans delayed non-COVID-19 healthcare treatments during the lockdowns. Two-thirds of that was considered necessary treatment. Probably the clearest data point that non-COVID-19 healthcare evaporated is in February 2020, healthcare spending was $1T (trillion!) more than April 2020. [176]

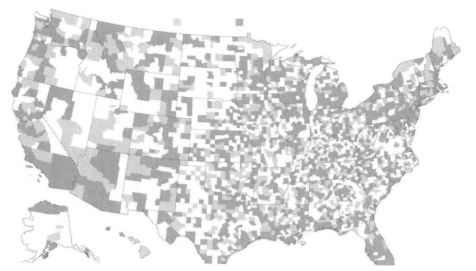

Hospital traffic compared to 2019: light grey: down 33-50%; dark grey: down 50% or more. 330

BUSINESSES LEAST AFFECTED

Not all companies realized economic downturns during the virus. Some would not just thrive but have some of their best performance ever. Netflix has 182 million subscribers and in the first quarter of 2020, they added 15 million subscribers, its best single quarter ever.[177] Disney Plus and Hulu saw growth during the shutdowns too. With live sports cancelled, the streaming services were a huge outlet for those seeking an escape. Microsoft's earnings and stock price jumped 15% with cloud usage and gaming up in the Spring of 2020.

Walgreens and CVS, both essential businesses, hired during the whole shutdown and fared well. Costco, Kroger and other similar essential businesses all saw spikes in sales as consumers stayed in, ate in, and binged on stocking up. Makers of constantly sold out items like toilet paper and paper towels saw record months. Costco's biggest inhibitor was inventory. During the lockdowns, Costco limited purchases of things like paper towels and toilet paper, and in May, would ration meats like beef, poultry and pork.

Amazon reached an incredible 2.54 billion visitors in March 2020, a 65% increase over March 2019.[178] Amazon has 40% of all online retail sales and half of the households in America have Amazon Prime accounts. Between entertainment and shopping for nonessential products sold, not to mention the convenience of free and quick shipping, Amazon was a winner out of the lockdowns.

The Great Depression of 1929 and the Great Recession of 2008 were both byproducts of lending practices, accidental happenings caused by bad policies. The economic collapse of 2020 was a forced occurrence, like a chain saw cutting the big Ohio oak tree in movie, *The Shawshank Redemption*. The strongest economy America had seen in decades was cut down by politicians and forced to her knees.

CHAPTER 12

MONEYBALL

The Major League Baseball season is opening up and they are instituting a new home run rule. Instead of requiring a ball to leave the ballpark in fair territory to qualify as a home run, they are expanding the rules. Now, as long as a ball is hit with a certain trajectory and exit velocity, it would be counted as a home run. It doesn't matter anymore if it leaves the ballpark. If it looked like it should be a home run, it would be counted.

Another interesting thing happened on Opening Day. Future Hall of Famer Justin Verlander pitched that first game for the Houston Astros. He got shelled in his first outing, giving up nine runs in three innings, ballooning his earned run average to 27.00. He was benched for months after that. It didn't matter that this was just one bad outing against a career ERA of 3.33 and an Astros career ERA of about 2.50. Verlander sat on the bench itching to get back on the mound but because of the one bad opening day performance, his coach sat him out in fear of another bad outing. His track record didn't matter.

Those two things did not actually happen, but similar things did happen in the data analytics of COVID-19. We began counting COVID-19 deaths whether they left the ballpark or not (whether they were real causes or not). And, like Verlander's bad outing, the breakout in New York shellshocked America into fear of another bad outing, thus putting Americans on the bench for much of 2020. If you watched television news, read the newspaper, visited online news sites or read social media, it was hard to understand what really happened.

The CDC counted anyone that died with COVID-19 as a COVID-19 death, even if that was not the *cause* of death. Then they counted anyone who *may* have had COVID-19 as a COVID-19 death. Given the overlap of deaths with other diseases like the flu and pneumonia, or cancer, or a car accident in one California case, all of which were counted as COVID-19 deaths as long as they carried the virus, the only way to measure the real impact COVID-19 had on America and the world is to look at all-cause mortalities year-over-year.

Without a doubt, deaths went up in March and April 2020 in many states. When 2020 conclusive data is available for all-cause mortality death increases in America, it may end up close to zero. On a two-year average into 2022, given the lives COVID-19 claimed, there is no doubt more increases in all-cause mortality will come from unchecked non-COVID-19 ailments and deaths of despair than COVID-19.

If COVID-19 does increase all-cause deaths over CDC expectations, it will likely not conclude more than a few percentage points up given in May 2020 the United States was 2% *below* year-to-date expected deaths for 2020.[179] In mid-June it was up 3% but fluctuating every day.

After all that data is analyzed, we know the data reporting on COVID-19 deaths is not clean, but directionally accurate. Here are the variable considerations on the reported COVID-19 deaths reliability of accuracy and how they may raise or lower *actual* COVID-19-caused fatalities. The net is a high probability that COVID-19 deaths were overstated due to other conditions or inflictions.

Unreported COVID-19 deaths	↑
Counting "probable COVID-19 deaths	↓
Lower than usual classified influenza deaths	↓
Lower than usual classified pneumonia deaths	↓
COVID-19 positive deaths by other causes (like a car crash)	↓
Other comorbidities not counted as cause of death	↓

The following chapters examine how COVID-19 deaths were undercounted, overcounted, the effects of all-cause mortality, who was dying and what happened in states and other countries.

CHAPTER 13

OVERCOUNTING AND UNDERCOUNTING FATALITIES

OVERCOUNTING FATALITIES

At the time of the lockdowns beginning March 19, 2020 in California and followed by most states within 10 days, the projection of American deaths was 2.2MM lives lost by August 2020. On that date, the Imperial College model was the standard. By March 26, the projection of lives lost was down to 150,000 to 200,000. Within days the estimation dropped from the IHME model to a range of 38,000 to 162,000. At this point, states locked down, millions lost their jobs, schools were closed and hundreds of millions of Americans stayed at home.

Would governors have closed their states if the fatality projections were two times 2017-2018 flu deaths? State governments were the authorities to lock down and reopen their states, not the federal government. With lost jobs, schools closed, empty hospitals and deaths not coming close to projections, we saw the counting of COVID-19 fatalities change. The counting of COVID-19 fatalities went from positive COVID-19 tests in those who died to those who died with a probability they had COVID-19.

By doing that, the fatality counts elevated and therefore inched closer to the projections that prompted the economic and social shutdowns. On the other side of the death equation, many cities reported they experienced higher than average deaths in homes, suggesting many people died with COVID-19 who were not tested nor hospitalized, a very reasonable assertion.

Another factor muddying the data is counting people who died *with* COVID-19 rather than *from* COVID-19. In the end, the most accurate data is looking at year-over-year all-cause mortalities in 2020 compared to 2019, as well as CDC reporting on where the country landed compared to expected deaths for 2020.

CDC GUIDELINES

In a March 24 memo, the CDC called for this in its directive to healthcare providers classifying COVID-19 deaths:

> *"Will COVID-19 be the underlying cause? The underlying cause depends upon what and where conditions are reported on the death certificate. However, the rules for coding and selection of the underlying cause of death are expected to result in COVID19 being the underlying cause more often than not.*
>
> *Should 'COVID-19' be reported on the death certificate only with a confirmed test? COVID-19 should be reported on the death certificate for all decedents where the disease caused or is assumed to have caused or contributed to death. Certifiers should include as much detail as possible based on their knowledge of the case, medical records, laboratory testing, etc. If the decedent had other chronic conditions such as COPD or asthma that may have also contributed, these conditions can be reported in Part II."*[180]

The CDC included probable deaths in the official death count total. As Georgia began reopening on April 24, the death total in the U.S. was 52,459 and this included 5,402 probable deaths.[181]

The New York Times reported on April 14 that "'Three thousand more people died in New York City between March 11 and April 13 than would have been expected during the same time period in an ordinary year,' Dr. Oxiris Barbot, the commissioner of the city Health Department, said in an interview."[182] Dr. Barbot is saying that, at that time, New York was up 3,000 all-cause deaths year-over-year while New York was reporting more than 10,000 COVID-19 deaths.[183]

On April 13, New York state reported more than 3,700 COVID-19 fatalities for that day, which was elevated with victims who did not test positive for COVID-19 but were presumed to have died with it over the previous month. Their otherwise highest reported fatality day was a fifth of that. This inclusion bumped up the total number of New York fatalities and it grew the United States total 17% increase, all in one day.

Can you see how the data loses some integrity and you aren't really sure what the real numbers are? Dr. Barbot raised an excellent statistic in identifying that New York was a net 3,000 up in deaths in the same period compared to more than three times that in COVID-19 deaths. In the All-Cause chapter, you will see how this cannibalized usual deaths of other causes. When this is all over in each country, when factoring in age and life expectancy, pre-existing conditions, flu and pneumonia and other deaths that would be undercounted and similar overlaps, comparing year-over-year all-cause mortality is the only way to evaluate the impact of COVID-19.

On May 11, *The Washington Post* reported that Dr. Deborah Birx felt the CDC was using methods of tracking that may be inflating the COVID-19 fatality counts by as much as 25%. "*There is nothing from the CDC that I can trust,*" Birx reportedly said, according to two of the Post's sources. It's a very indicting comment coming from maybe the number two medical expert leading the COVID-19 response from the federal government.

Dr. Scott Jensen is a Minnesota physician and a state senator. He gave an example of a patient who died while having the flu. Jensen said typically if the patient had symptoms like a fever and cough (flu-like symptoms), he would code the death as "*respiratory arrest. I've never been encouraged to [notate 'influenza']. I would probably write 'respiratory arrest' to be the top line, and the underlying cause of this disease would be pneumonia ... I might well put emphysema or congestive heart failure, but I would never put influenza down as the underlying cause of death and yet that's what we are being asked to do here.*"

Jensen then told the interviewer that under the CDC guidelines, a patient who died after being hit by a bus and tested positive for coronavirus would be listed as a COVID-19 death, regardless of whatever damage was caused by the bus. Further, he called out "*Right now Medicare has determined that if you have a COVID-19 admission to the hospital you'll get paid $13,000 [compared to a standard $5,000]. If that COVID-19 patient goes on a ventilator, you get $39,000; three times as much. Nobody can tell me, after 35 years in the world of medicine, that sometimes those kinds of things [have] impact on what we do.*"[184]

The CARES Act government bailout initiative paid by another estimate a 20% increase in Medicare reimbursements for COVID-19 hospitalizations. The add-on was authorized by the coronavirus stimulus package signed into law on March 27.[185]

Revcycle Intelligence noted that even with higher payouts for COVID-19 patients, the costs associated with treatments are greater, in which case hospitals would lose money overall per patient.[186] In speaking with several physicians, they all doubted hospitals were changing death classifications for financial gain.

PENNSYLVANIA

Pennsylvania followed New York's lead and began including "probable" COVID-19 deaths in their count around April 21. That resulted in ballooning their total death count by nearly double in a couple of days. After some scrutiny and criticism, the Pennsylvania Department of Health (DOH) backtracked and removed the "probables" in their tally.[187]

None of these dirty data observations is meant to suggest that COVID-19 was not a real health event. It was and spending any time in New York or Detroit in early April illuminated that. Data integrity inspires confidence and adjusting death counts by 10% or 20% doesn't change the bigger picture of the virus' effect.

With deaths and hospitalizations so much lower than projections and when profiling the victims, no amount of data inflation was going to justify the social and economic lockdowns across the country and world.

COLORADO

If you think government agencies would not try to overcount COVID-19 fatalities, consider what happened in Colorado at the end of April 2020. The Colorado Department of Public Health and Environment reclassified three deaths at a Centennial nursing home as COVID-19 deaths. Attending physicians ruled all three were not related to coronavirus, and yet their cause of death was overridden.[188]

The unsettling part of this is that, eventually, stories like this always come out. Data integrity is everything for citizens to have confidence in their government, health organizations and the media. Why overstate the COVID-19 deaths? The best news everyone can get is that we dodged one, and that the coronavirus pandemic was less dangerous than anyone thought. The problem is that would require most health and government officials to admit the lockdowns were overblown, with 40 million jobs lost and the greatest domestic crisis in American history since the Civil War and with the Great Depression.

Steven Schwartz is the Director of Vital Statistics at the CDC. On March 4, he sent a memo to hospital administrators advising them to code COVID-19 as the cause of death if it was the known cause or likely cause of death. On March 24, he sent another note guiding administrators that COVID-19 is expected to more often than not be the cause of death, regardless if the patient has underlying conditions such as COPD or asthma.

Given the policy making and public concern for real data, the guidance should have been something like, "If you code a cause of death to COVID-19, it should be verified that both the patient tested positive for the virus and you concluded it was the primary cause of death." Otherwise, the integrity of the data is fractured.

On May 13, near Durango, CO, another controversy erupted because a 35-year-old man died from alcohol poisoning, with a .55% blood-alcohol level, seven times the legal limit. In the autopsy, the man tested positive for COVID-19 and was counted as a COVID-19 death. Should this be counted as a COVID-19 death, if he died with it but not from it?[189]

If he died with HIV but from a car crash, is it a HIV death? These may be outliers, but they're the ones we heard about. If tens of millions of people had COVID-19 or the antibodies by summer, entirely possible, then many deaths could be COVID-19 deaths. This makes comparing all-cause mortality deaths to prior years to only reliable metric left to determine the impact of the virus. It's the one metric not manipulated.

On May 15, Colorado began to change their coding of COVID-19 deaths, breaking it up into people who died *from* COVID-19 and people who died *with* COVID-19. In one day, the state's COVID-19 fatalities dropped 25%. Does anyone else see how fast this was moving and how, under scrutiny, we started to get cleaner data? Apply that ratio to the country total and we're 25% under the bad flu season two years earlier at the time of the re-openings. That's without any lockdowns, lost jobs, closed schools or a shutdown healthcare system.

The next day, Colorado Governor Jared Polis, a Democrat, blasted the way the CDC was counting COVID-19 deaths as it was not reflecting accurately who was dying from the illness. He pointed to the Durango alcohol poisoning death and called it a point of reckoning. Polis would be on his way to reelection.

UNDERCOUNTING FATALITIES

While overcounting fatalities was uncovered with hard data, other data suggested that early (February and March) COVID-19 deaths were undercounted and probably by a high number. The challenge with analyzing these deaths, and even those caused by the flu is, did the patient die with the virus or because of the virus?

Two things could account for this. First, the patient died from COVID-19 but was not tested. Second, they died from something else because they did not get normal health care for their ailment because either they could not get in to see their healthcare provider or they were afraid to do so for fear of catching COVID-19.

Below is a terrific graphic provided by the Gothamist. They charted New York City deaths in the home in this period. On average, that number is about 25 per day, and you can see the huge increase for a period of days in New York. Those deaths may or may not have been due to COVID-19, but the dots sure connect increased deaths in the home to the timing of the COVID-19 break-out there.

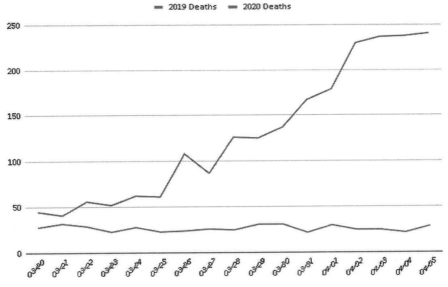

Source: https://gothamist.com/news/death-count-expected-soar-nyc-says-it-will-begin-reporting-suspected-covid-deaths-addition-confirmed-ones

While the premise in this book is that the actual COVID-19 deaths never war-ranted the models, nor the economic and social lockdowns, there's little doubt the *actual* deaths with COVID-19 could be higher than those reported, perhaps by 10-15%, from fatalities that occurred in February and March. It's doubtful they were undercounted from April on because probables became included, as well as so much attention brought to all death classifications. However, it's then lower than reported because many died *with* COVID-19 but not *from* it.

CHAPTER 14

NURSING HOMES

Nursing home residents proved to be most vulnerable to COVID-19. It became the hotbed for the virus spread and the source of most deaths. In Europe, it's estimated more than half of the deaths were residents of long-term-care facilities.[190] In America, the data is not tied together in one data source like the CDC (yet), but it's significant and likely to be well over 50% of all COVID-19 deaths too (officially at 43% in June but many states are not reporting). Below is some reporting on the impact on people living in long term care facilities:

- *"70% of Ohio coronavirus deaths have occurred in long-term care facilities"* [191]
- *"One-Third of All U.S. Coronavirus Deaths Are Nursing Home Residents or Workers; At least 25,600 residents and workers have died from the coronavirus at nursing homes and other long-term care facilities for older adults in the United States. The virus so far has infected more than 143,000 at some 7,500 facilities."*[192] *That number would jump substantially as more data came in.*
- *"Nearly 50% of California's COVID-19 deaths are residents, staff at nursing, care homes"*[193]
- *"Nursing homes account for 48% of all Illinois COVID-19 deaths"*[194]
- *"70% of Johnson County (southern part of metro Kansas City, KS) deaths were in at least eight different long-term care facilities"*[195]
- *"Elder Care Facilities In Mass. The Hardest, With More Than 1,300 Now Dead."*[196] *Massachusetts had just over 3,000 COVID-19 deaths at the end of April*
- *"Nursing homes account for one-third of Indiana coronavirus deaths"*[197]
- *"The deaths of 322 residents of nursing homes and senior care centers in Colorado have been linked to COVID-19."* *Colorado had just over 700 COVID-19 deaths at the end of April 2020.*[198]

- *"A quarter of the deaths in Queens and Brooklyn came from nursing homes and adult care facilities."[199]*
- *"40% of the COVID-19 deaths in Georgia were in long-term care facilities, including nursing homes, according to data from the Georgia Department of Community Health (DCH) and the Georgia Department of Public Health (DPH)."[200]*
- *"Louisiana has had 275 COVID-19 deaths among residents at long term care facilities, and about 1,100 at the end of April."[201]*
- *"The WHO reported nursing homes linked to up to half of coronavirus deaths in Europe"[202]*
- *"In Michigan, more than 2,000 nursing home patients had COVID-19 at the end of April."[203]*
- *"Of Florida's first 1,074 COVID-19 deaths, 311 were long term care residents, almost a third. This was much less than some states like Delaware (58%), Massachusetts (55%) and Colorado (50%)."[204]*
- *"Coronavirus-linked fatalities at nursing homes and other long-term care facilities in the US have surpassed 10,000 — with the highest tally in New York. A survey by the Wall Street Journal published Wednesday found at least 10,700 fatalities among 35 states that either submit data online or responded to information requests."[205]*
- *"Nearly 60 percent of Virginia's coronavirus deaths are in nursing homes, other long-term care facilities."[206] In the first week of May, more deaths were counted in nursing homes than overall COVID-19 totals in Maryland and Virginia, which meant not only were all the fatalities coming from nursing homes, but they were backdating. Nothing wrong with that, other than schools remained closed and people remained locked down with all the risk narrowed to one segment of the population.*
- *"Over 40% of Texas deaths were linked to nursing homes and long-term care facilities."[207]*
- *"68% of Pennsylvania's 3,106 COVID-19 deaths by early May were sourced from nursing homes and related facilities."[208]*
- *"Minnesota nursing homes, already the site of 81% of COVID-19 deaths, continue taking in infected patients."[209]*
- *"U.S. Nursing Homes Have More Coronavirus Deaths Than All But 5 Countries, and the Counting Has Just Begun."[210]*
- *"Canada's nursing home crisis: 81 percent of coronavirus deaths are in long-term care facilities"[211]*
- New York, New Jersey and California each had policies in April requiring nursing homes to admit patients deemed stable but with COVID-19.

Stable patients would surely enjoy time in a nursing home more than a hospital. A criteria set was that staff and patients would be careful not to comingle the patients and staff would be tested but based on reports that seemed difficult and inconsistent. At a glance, this appears to be one of the stranger policies to enact – placing the most vulnerable infected people in a dwelling with the most vulnerable non-infected people.[212]

While not-at-risk citizens were locked down, the majority of real at-risk people were dying at a slow but steady pace because they started the first two months of the pandemic unprotected in most places. More than 60% of the deaths in Ohio, Pennsylvania, Minnesota, Massachusetts, New Jersey and Connecticut were nursing home patients, and in neighboring Rhode Island it was more like 70%. More people died in nursing homes by a factor of more than 60% than all other deaths in Connecticut combined.

Below is a visual of the percent of nursing home deaths in states as of early May. Some states do not have crisp reporting data, and New York is undercounted based on its reporting.

Share of COVID-19 Deaths Occurring in Nursing & Assisted Living Facilities
(Based on Data Reported by June 14, 2020)

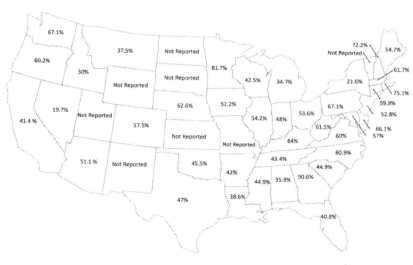

Each state is reporting through state sites linked from the AARP site here: https://www.aarp.org/caregiving/health/info-2020/coronavirus-nursing-home-cases-deaths.html

We will never know exactly the number of COVID-19 deaths that occurred in care facilities or were sourced there, but it's sad when you think of inconsistent care and the immobility of the residents. One woman lost her grandfather, a World War II veteran, to COVID-19 in a nursing home. She said that the residents were "sitting ducks" as this swept through his nursing home.

Many states and nursing homes are not required to release this data and are not motivated to do so. Several states are indemnifying care facilities and their employees (who may have been sources of the spread), and many more are requesting their states to do so. This will grow into 2020 and 2021 and there will likely be a storm of wrongful death lawsuits against facilities and employees. If states do not indemnify nursing homes, many less will exist by 2021.

Still, the early data showed that while the general populace was at very low risk, thus never justifying the social and economic lockdowns, few analyzed the data to put military-like protections and testing in place at these facilities.

MOST FLAWED POLICY

There are many variables to consider when looking at the fatalities in a short-term view but consider two different approaches to navigating the pandemic. Early on, New York state mandated their long-term and associated care facilities admit patients with COVID-19. So did California. Florida mandated early on that no patient could enter a care facility unless they tested negative for the virus. Two different approaches, two different outcomes.

Now, had Governor Cuomo done what Governor DeSantis did, New York would still have had the highest deaths in the world per capita, but it would have been better. For all the policy decisions made by state and federal governments, wasn't this the most reckless? If we knew one thing by early March, it's that the elderly were the most vulnerable. What kind of thoughtless policy went into requiring infected patients be co-mingled with the most vulnerable? Where were the medical experts on the front end of this?

We did a good job of locking down all demographics equally, and uselessly, but did a poor job of surgically protecting those most likely to fall victim to COVID-19. It was the single worst policy move any state or federal leader would make.

By the end of May, this policy flaw was highlighted by many in the media, but the blame was placed on politicians. You have to imagine for a moment what was likely going on in those war rooms. Governor Cuomo sitting with his team, including perhaps someone from the CDC and state health services. He's asking them for advice, as did most governors. They didn't call out the risk, and as experts in the field with the data we knew then, they should have. From healthcare counsel to the WHO to the CDC to state health leaders, they failed to see what was in front of them, prompting awful policies issued by our leaders.

INTERNATIONAL

In Ontario, Canada, 70% of the COVID-19 deaths came from care homes. Across Canada, the British Columbia Centre for Disease Control reported a total of 112 deaths as a result of COVID-19, of which 70 (63%) were patients/residents in care facilities, which includes acute care institutions, long-term care homes, assisted and independent living establishments.[213]

Around 53% of all COVID-19 victims in Belgium died in care homes. Sciensano, a public research institute, reported of the total deaths, 83% of all-care-home deaths were suspected cases. The report also contained data on the number of care-home staff and residents who have been tested since April 10.

As of May 3, 88,883 staff were tested. Of these, 3% were positive, and of those who tested positive, 72% were asymptomatic. Of the 68,336 residents who had been tested, 7% were positive and of these, 74% were asymptomatic.[214]

The data from France was inconsistent but on the high-end estimate, more than 50% of the COVID-19 victims were sourced from long-term-care facilities and on the low end, more than 40%. While Germany was less affected than many peers in the EU, up to half of their COVID-19 deaths were sourced from nursing homes.

The first COVID-19 case in Italy was on January 30. The average age of COVID-19 deaths was 79 in Italy and the median was 81. The largest nursing home in Italy became subject to lawsuits by the families of victims, where that home had a 61% increase in deaths in the first half of 2020 compared to a five-year average. The exact percent of nursing home deaths compared to all COVID-19 deaths in Italy is still unclear, early data suggests about 50%.

We were lucky on the front end of the pandemic to know who was most vulnerable. Most states, our country and the world as a whole did a poor job protecting and isolating this segment of the population.

CHAPTER 15

ALL-CAUSE MORTALITY IN AMERICA

medRxiv reported this commentary on the accuracy of counting COVID-19 deaths:

> *"Deaths attributed to COVID-19 are also difficult to measure accurately. Problems with testing affect not only confirmed cases but also attributed deaths. Besides, testing is not enough to determine the cause of death, as some patients may die while infected with SARS-CoV-2, but not due to it. Due to constraints health systems are facing across the world, it is likely that a precise attribution of cause of death is not possible. Additionally, some patients die without there having been a suspicion of COVID19."[215]*

The United States loses almost 8,000 people on average every day. With muddy COVID-19 fatality data, the best way to determine COVID-19's impact is to compare year-over-year all-cause mortality deaths. This takes the 3,000,000 people who died in America on average between 2015-2017 and compares that to the number of people who died in 2020, regardless why they died. First, *figure 1* is a chart illustrating some scale between COVID-19 deaths and all deaths in America:

Of the 857,948 deaths in America in the three-plus-month period, COVID-19 deaths are about 7% of that total. On average we lose 50,000 people per year to pneumonia, more than a million people to cardiovascular diseases and 83,000 to diabetes, all causes that COVID-19 would exploit. This is just to provide scale to COVID-19 in 2020. COVID-19 did cause incremental deaths, but others listed decreased some as the cause of comorbidities with COVID-19 were coded as COVID-19 deaths.

Figure 2 shows average daily deaths from the flu in 2019, about 34,000 deaths in seven months. The data for the COVID-19 deaths is an average from February 15

Figure 1

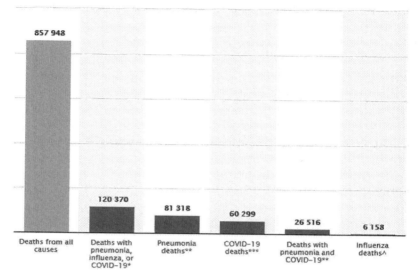

Number of deaths involving coronavirus disease 2019 (COVID-19), pneumonia, and influenza in the U.S. from February 1 to May 9, 2020.
Source: https://www.statista.com/statistics/1113051/number-reported-deaths-from-covid-pneumonia-and-flu-us/

Figure 2

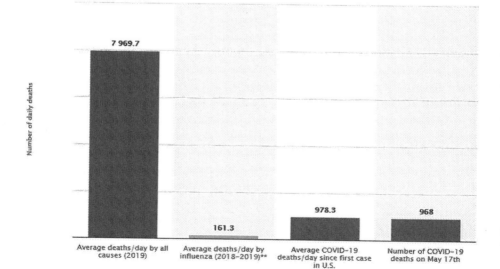

Source: https://www.statista.com/statistics/1109281/covid-19-daily-deaths-compared-to-all-causes/

through May 18. The COVID-19 timeframe is compressed, of course, but no matter how you read this, COVID-19 was bigger than the flu the year before.

Below is a CDC chart identifying all-cause deaths in America from February – May 18, 2020, as well as those with COVID-19 and related causes of death. Of the 876,866 deaths in America that occurred between February through May 18, 2020, 97% were "expected." That leaves 27,000 fewer than "expected" deaths in this period. Read that again. After the height of the pandemic, we were below average in total deaths in the U.S.

The chart below is updated daily. On June 9, 2020, we were 102% of expected deaths, up about 20,000 over normal while we had recorded 114,000 COVID-19 deaths on this date. In late June that jumped to 106%. This is the most important statistic to follow to determine the COVID-19 impact.

Influenza deaths are listed at 6,180. A typical flu season from October through April any given year may kill from 30,000 to a high in 2017-2018 of 80,000 people. The peak month is almost always February, followed by January. The influenza deaths listed may have included patients with COVID-19 from the beginning of February. It's very likely that thousands of the COVID-19 deaths displaced deaths that would have been attributed to the flu.

MOST IMPORTANT METRIC

Updated May 18, 2020

Week ending date in which the death occurred	COVID-19 Deaths (U07.1)	Deaths from All Causes	Percent of Expected Deaths²	Pneumonia Deaths (J12.0-J18.9)³	Deaths with Pneumonia and COVID-19 (J12.0-J18.9 and U07.1)³	Influenza Deaths (J09-J11)⁴	Deaths with Pneumonia, Influenza, or COVID-19 (U07.1 or J09-J18.9)⁵
Total Deaths	62,515	876,866	97	83,333	27,542	6,180	123,593
2/1/2020	0	57,551	97	3,707	0	473	4,180
2/8/2020	1	58,151	97	3,706	0	507	4,214
2/15/2020	0	57,490	98	3,734	0	537	4,271
2/22/2020	2	57,527	99	3,603	0	553	4,158
2/29/2020	7	57,816	100	3,714	5	626	4,342
3/7/2020	32	57,408	99	3,799	16	608	4,422
3/14/2020	51	55,993	98	3,793	26	598	4,415
3/21/2020	517	56,213	99	4,309	237	521	5,104
3/28/2020	2,900	59,586	107	5,846	1,312	422	7,807
4/4/2020	8,921	67,586	121	9,270	4,278	445	14,138
4/11/2020	14,361	72,933	131	11,043	6,407	451	19,117
4/18/2020	14,243	68,528	127	9,985	6,149	247	18,145
4/25/2020	11,049	61,220	114	8,047	4,758	131	14,382
5/2/2020	7,069	49,828	92	5,528	2,961	46	9,666
5/9/2020	2,943	31,658	60	2,730	1,228	14	4,458
5/16/2020	419	7,378	14	519	165	1	774

Source: https://www.cdc.gov/nchs/nvss/vsrr/covid19/index.htm

The CDC also puts out data on "expected deaths" for the United States and each state, the fourth column above. Expected deaths "is the number of deaths for all causes in 2020 compared to the average number across the same [period] in 2017–2019." Below is how, according to the CDC, select states and the country fared at the height of the pandemic in expected death totals.[216] The context in the next chart is perhaps the most important in this book:

ALL-CAUSE MORTALITY IN AMERICA

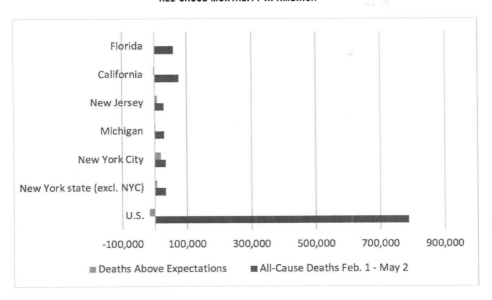

	ALL-CAUSE DEATHS FEB. 1 - MAY 18	DEATHS ABOVE EXPECTATIONS
U.S.	876,866	-27,120
New York state (excl. NYC)	35,024	6778
New York City	34,713	19620
Michigan	29,771	2706
New Jersey	29,326	8378
California	75,184	1534
Florida	59,149	0

All-cause deaths in America from February 1 through May 18, 2020 in the United States were on average below expectations based on CDC data. This is the time frame of the reopening debates. That rose later into May and June, but the point is to provide scale – how bad overall were death totals compared to expectations?

With 70,000 COVID-19 deaths recorded by this date, we can see the actual number of all deaths nationwide is below average. When we reached 120,000 in June we were above average by about 60,000. No doubt New York and New Jersey were way up, but overall, the country was about flat. For that we locked down 326,000,000 people, prompted 40 million to be unemployed, destroyed untold thousands of businesses, not to mention prompted other ailments to trigger deaths because they would go untreated and likely cause more deaths later in 2020 and into 2021.

The CDC states that their reported data could be off due to delayed reporting for up to eight weeks. Therefore, it's possible the 2020 actual data for all-cause deaths may be a little higher.

In reconciling the CDC data with the state of Michigan data for identical periods, the CDC reported all-cause deaths of this period at 29,771 where Michigan reported same period deaths at 27,872.[217] In this case, the CDC is higher, which makes one think the data is close to accurate. At the same time, consider that at this time, data and death reporting was hypersensitive, and given that attention it's likely more accurate than in non-emergency times.

What this shows is that from an all-cause mortality perspective at the end of April 2020:

- The United States was actually below expectations or flat in all deaths
- California was actually below expectations in all deaths
- New York City was more than twice as high as expected
- New York state, not counting New York City, was above expectations
- New Jersey was well above expectations
- Michigan was 10 percent more than expectations
- Florida was even and had the same number of deaths as expected

This data has to be contextualized. The political leaders made the decision to lock down nearly all states' citizens, force them to stay at home, close businesses and prompt 40 million people to lose their livelihoods. They refused to reopen the country while total death expectations through the end of the high point of the pandemic were essentially flat.

America loses 38,000 people a year to car deaths. COVID-19 put the entire population at about twice the risk, in absolute numbers, of dying as they would be of getting in the car to drive every year. If you isolate the vulnerable, those with the top five or six pre-existing conditions and very elderly, then the rest would be much less at risk of dying from COVID-19 than from driving, virtually no statistical risk. For that, would we really lock down the entire country, force 40 million Americans out of work, shut down schools, the entire healthcare system?

ALL-CAUSE MORTALITY IN AMERICA

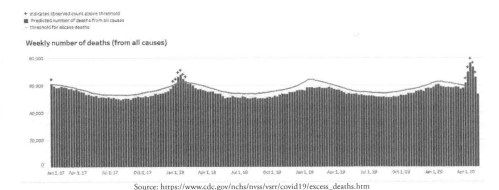

Source: https://www.cdc.gov/nchs/nvss/vsrr/covid19/excess_deaths.htm

The CDC chart above shows all deaths in the United States for the past three years. The yellow line is the threshold line for excess deaths in any period. Under that is considered normal. You can see the spike around the 2017-2018 flu season. What happened to the United States in 2020 was a below average number of deaths early in the year before the pandemic struck. It spiked sharply in late March and early April, then it settled back close to normal.

In Italy, you can see the same period 2019 compared to 2020 and the overall increase in deaths. Italy recorded 27,000 COVID-19 deaths in March and April 2020. When you reconcile that with the chart below, there's no doubt of COVID-19's impact.

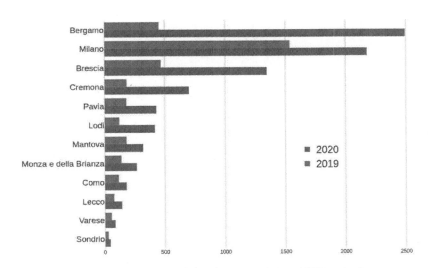

Deaths 1-21 / March - 2019 vs 2020 by Province

Source: https://towardsdatascience.com/covid-19-excess-mortality-figures-in-italy-d9640f411691

Interestingly, when reviewing excess mortality due to the flu in Italy in recent years, Science Direct performed the following analysis: "*We estimated excess deaths of 7,027, 20,259, 15,801 and 24,981 attributable to influenza epidemics in the 2013/14, 2014/15, 2015/16 and 2016/17, respectively, using the Goldstein index.*"[218] If you average the latter three seasons, you see 20,347 deaths above all-cause in those years.

Regardless, two things are clear: COVID-19 added to all-cause deaths in Italy and also displaced flu deaths that would have incrementally added to total deaths in the Winter and Spring of 2020.

European all-cause mortality data showed total deaths above average in nearly all western European countries.

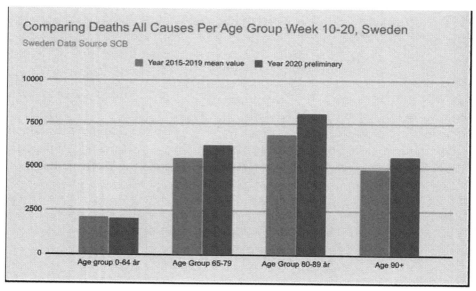

Source: https://www.scb.se/om-scb/nyheter-och-pressmeddelanden/scb-publicerar-preliminar-statistik-over-doda-i-sverige/

One final chart above. After 10 weeks of COVID-19 and no lockdowns, Sweden was actually below the all-cause mortality average for the age grouping below age 65, while up for the older age groups. This was no surprise considering the data from the cruise ships.

COVID-19 DATA ON FATALITIES

One consistent data point we learned from the cruise ships, the early breakout in Italy and all the data well-documented in America was that COVID-19 was a discriminating disease. Unlike the Spanish Flu or HIV, which killed a wide demographic of people of all ages and health conditions, COVID-19 proved to be most dangerous to the vulnerable: the elderly with frail immune systems, and nearly all other deaths in people suffering from chronic conditions. Of patients hospitalized the breakdown in underlying conditions was:

Obesity	48.3%
Diabetes	28.3%
Serious heart conditions	27.8%
Hypertension	49.7%
Chronic lung disease	34.6%

Source: https://www.cdc.gov/coronavirus/2019-ncov/need-extra-precautions/groups-at-higher-risk.html

Through the first 80,000 COVID-19 deaths in America, below are the number of patients that had the following underlying conditions. Many had more than one, so these are not mutually exclusive to each other. The point here is we have the ability to identify and isolate the most vulnerable with some precision.

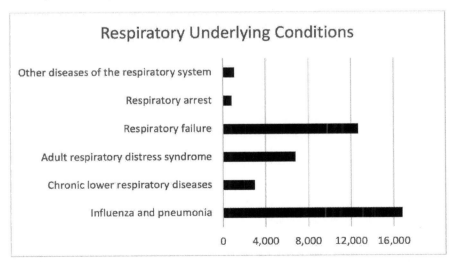

Source: CDC https://data.cdc.gov/NCHS/Conditions-contributing-to-deaths-involving-corona/hk9y-quqm/data

179

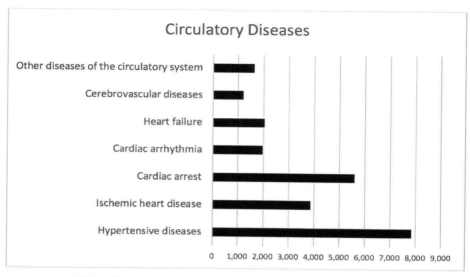

Source: CDC https://data.cdc.gov/NCHS/Conditions-contributing-to-deaths-involving-corona/hk9y-quqm/data

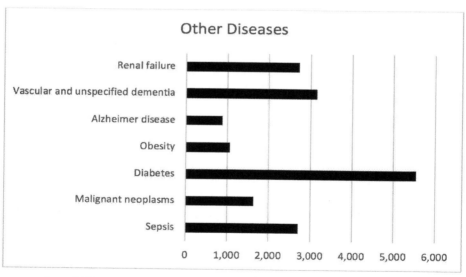

Source: CDC https://data.cdc.gov/NCHS/Conditions-contributing-to-deaths-involving-corona/hk9y-quqm/data

A *Reuters* article stated that "some 97% of those killed by COVID-19 in Louisiana had a pre-existing condition, according to the state health department. Diabetes was seen in 40% of the deaths, obesity in 25%, chronic kidney disease in 23% and cardiac problems in 21%."[219]

OBESITY

Below is a chart mapping obesity percentages of the population in each country. It's interesting that two of the wealthiest countries on the globe are darkest blue. And, save for China, since we have not been able to rely on COVID-19 data from there, lighter colors resulted in fewer COVID-19 effects, except for Italy and Spain. And, with the exception of Japan and South Korea, you can see a correlation between obesity and wealthier nations.

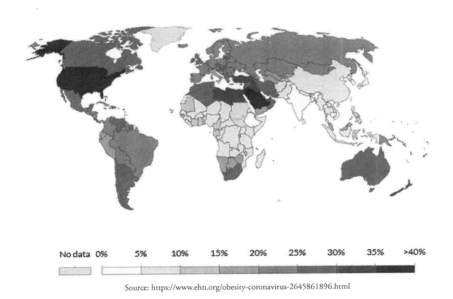

Source: https://www.ehn.org/obesity-coronavirus-2645861896.html

As part of the COVID-19 response team at O'Connor Hospital in San Jose, Calif., Nivedita Lakhera wasn't prepared to see her intensive care unit filled with so many young patients. Many of those patients had no medical condition other than obesity. "They are young and coming to the ER and just dropping dead," she says. Some doctors say that some of their sickest patients are those under 60 who are obese.[220]

America has one of the highest obesity rates in the world. Obesity was the number one underlying condition causing death from COVID-19 in victims under age 65. In the United States, more than 40% of adults have a body mass index (BMI) greater than 30, the threshold for obesity. Nearly 10% are "severely obese" if they have a BMI greater than 40, according to the CDC.

What is obesity? Below is a BMI chart. In reviewing it, the beginning of the yellow (overweight) boxes fringe on what would be normal. For myself, I fell into the last "normal" box on a row and feel I need to put on some weight. My son, a D1 athlete in college has 3% body fat and he too is on the last "normal" box on his row.

About 40% of Americans are in the obese or extremely obese boxes on the chart. When I mentioned that data to many of the physicians with whom I spoke with in researching this book, each rolled their eyes at me and shook their heads; they knew. That's with many of them falling into those same right-hand boxes by their own admission.

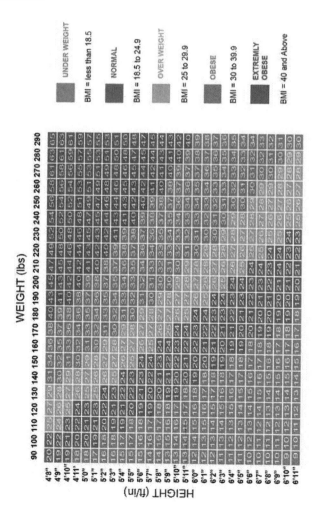

COVID-19 was causing strokes at a much higher than usual rate in people under 50 who were obese. Usually strokes occur from blood clots in arteries, but doctors were seeing clots in veins in COVID-19 patients.[221]

The United States loses more than 80,000 people to diabetes any given year.[222] If we are able to in the future see the combination of diabetes deaths with and without COVID-19, it is highly likely that number will be more than 100,000 in 2020.

The United States had 876,866 deaths in this period. Here is additional context:

- 123,593 people died with either pneumonia, the flu or COVID-19 or a combination, 14% of all deaths. In 2019, somewhere between 34,000 and over 50,000 people died from the flu. It's very likely there is overlap where otherwise flu-deaths became COVID-19 deaths.
- About half of the people who were hospitalized with COVID-19 were obese.[223] With the very low obesity rates in Japan and South Korea and India, this would account for their much lower level of inflictions.
- Pneumonia has been in close alignment and overlap with COVID-19 causes of death.

In one analysis, pneumonia deaths dropped off during the COVID-19 peak and appeared to displace them as a cause of death:

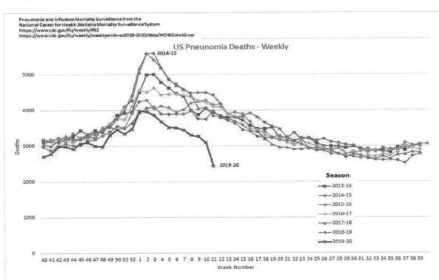

Source: https://skeptics.stackexchange.com/questions/47265/has-the-number-of-pneumonia-deaths-in-the-us-dramatically-dropped-in-2020

Based on this, it seems logical that a few thousand COVID-19 deaths would probably have occurred with pneumonia as a cause of death.

Below is the age distribution of COVID-19 deaths in the United States through April 2020. As of May 1, with extensive analysis of three continents (Australia, Europe and North America), not a single case of a child passing the virus on to an adult was found and no more than a handful of children died from it, and in those who did, the details were unclear if they had underlying conditions. Still, schools were closed and children's activities cancelled.

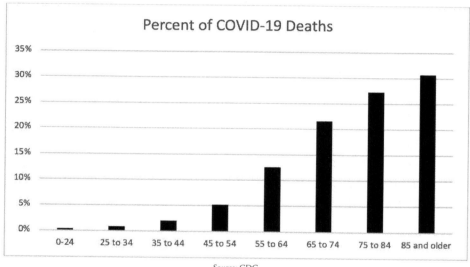

Source: CDC

Finally, look at the chart across the page illustrating the displacement of cause of deaths in New York state for this period. This should leave little doubt while some COVID-19 deaths were not counted, more were overcounted.

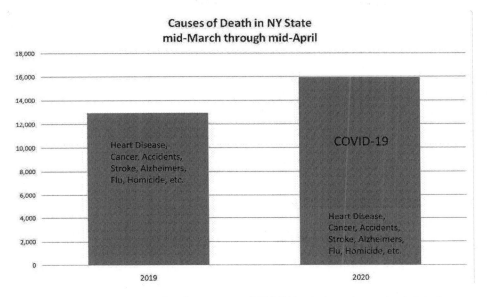

Source: CDC NY mortality stats & https://www.nytimes.com/2020/04/14/nyregion/new-york-coronavirus-deaths.html

In New York City, 89% of the COVID-19 deaths had at least one comorbidity.[224] In reviewing the data specifically, practically everyone who died between ages 30 and 60 had one or more of nine different comorbidities.

MICHIGAN

It's interesting in poring through data from state-to-state how each one reports, some with excellent analytics. Some states make it more challenging to understand what was happening between peak and total hospitalizations and COVID-19 deaths. It's also challenging to find COVID-19 deaths compared to other death causes in a year-over-year context. Michigan produced an informative report doing just that.

In March and April 2019, Michigan had 16,569 all-cause deaths. In March and April 2020, Michigan had 19,684 all-cause deaths, a difference of 3,115. By May 5, Michigan recorded 4,102 COVID-19 deaths. The COVID-19 deaths in the Michigan table below show a lower number than the "official" COVID-19 deaths you see in other sources like Worldometers or the CDC. Forget that for a moment, the data and reporting was happening fast and the point here is not that but comparing all-cause and specific causes in the comparison.[225]

The 2019 all-cause death comparisons to 2020 are close enough to fully believe and have confidence that the incremental deaths in Michigan were prompted by COVID-19. Also, when any argument is made that there is "massive" COVID-19 death under-counting, the data does not support undercounts. It looks very reasonable; it all adds up. Michigan's population of 10 million people had an increase of 3,115 all-cause deaths, representing .03% of the population. This is through April 2020. If the all-cause deaths double later into 2020 (to 6,230), the all-cause increase could grow to .06%.

Number of Deaths by Select Causes of Death by Month, Michigan Occurences, January, 01 2020—May 5, 2020[P]

Year of Death	Month of Death	Total	Cancer	Heart Disease	COPD	Stroke	Pneumonia & Flu	Septicemia	COVID-19
2019	January	8,490	797	2,273	486	441	176	108	–
2019	February	7,712	665	2,063	452	386	144	93	–
2019	March	8,582	775	2,230	522	476	197	87	–
2019	April	7,987	718	1,984	510	419	203	116	–
2019	May	8,163	794	2,090	486	418	140	78	–
2019	June	7,710	726	1,970	468	372	116	89	–
2019	July	7,992	835	1,998	456	412	109	93	–
2019	August	7,810	793	1,946	431	401	89	93	–
2019	September	7,733	767	1,883	444	405	109	87	–
2019	October	8,289	861	2,108	472	445	100	87	–
2019	November	8,391	726	2,191	462	421	121	106	–
2019	December	8,768	850	2,377	511	471	136	95	–
2020	January	8,915	855	2,219	603	513	180	116	–
2020	February	8,188	703	2,106	493	475	218	110	–
2020	March	9,354	796	2,268	569	477	302	119	387
2020	April	10,330	572	1,794	394	403	249	82	2,386
2020	May	7	–	–	–	–	–	–	1

Remember the initial models driving the lockdown suggested death rates of 1-7%. Even at 1%, Michigan would realize an increase in all-cause deaths due to COVID-19 of 100,000 people, and at 7%, 700,000 deaths.

- Michigan locked down with a presumption that on the low side 70,000 people would die from COVID -19
- After six weeks of lockdown, they had lost 3,115 more people than the previous year, two months into the pandemic

- If that doubled, they'd be at 10% of those projected losses, which means it's impossible they would near the projection that prompted the lockdown
- Michigan was the fourth most impacted state in the country, which means 46 other states were faring between better and much better
- With this data, Michigan continued to lock down into July and the economy restrained

Michigan was the hardest-hit state of any during the Great Depression. Auto sales dropped to just 25% of pre-depression sales. The only thing that pulled them out was the conversion of auto plants to make airplanes, ammunition, bombs and other supplies for the Allied forces in World War II. Michigan workers suffered greatly with the influx of foreign cars and automated manufacturing ever since the 1980s. The last thing Michigan needed was an economic closing to set back the progress they'd made in recent years. Still, the lockdown went on.

HOW LETHAL IS COVID-19?

The short answer is no one knows for sure. The longer answer is we have many data points to provide good direction on how bad this could get and who is vulnerable. One metric used for virus lethality is the infection fatality rate. If 1,000,000 people contract a virus and 100,000 die from it, the fatality rate is 10%, which is very high. If you look at the official numbers in the spring of 2020 on COVID-19, as of June 15, you see something close to 2,000,000 official cases and 100,000 deaths, a 5% fatality rate, also very high.

However, many more people contracted the virus and were not sick at all or only mildly sick, in which case they were not tested. Based on case studies we will see in the next chapter, it could be many times the official case totals. If we have 2,000,000 official cases, it's not a leap to imagine 50 million or more have contracted SARS-CoV-2. That's a twenty-five-fold increase and case studies have suggested that, some more than that.

Seroprevalence in this case is the frequency of SARS-CoV-2 in the population. A *medRxiv* study estimated in June 2020 a range of .1% to 47%,[226] an enormous range of possible exposure. In the United States, that equates to a range of 326,000 to 153,000,000 people. We know that the official count is more than two million and based on case studies, much higher.

An infection fatality rate (IFR) is the death rate among those infected, not the entire population. They went on to estimate an IFR of .02% to .86% on the population as a whole. Among people under 70, they estimated an IFR of .0% to .26%. For context, a typical flu IFR might be .05% depending on the season. This places COVID-19 less lethal than the flu for those under 70 and more lethal than the flu for those over 70. The hard data we have discussed here supports those conclusions.

CHAPTER 16

CASES, CASES, CASES!

By April 27, 2020, Texas and Georgia were leading the way with reopening their economies and social options. With the second largest economy in the United States in Texas, there was little doubt most states would follow quickly. The initial crisis we faced with COVID-19 was not having enough hospital capacity. When that never happened (we never got to full capacity, even in New York City), the argument for and against reopening states became all about cases and testing.

Cases became a very controversial data point as states would begin to reopen. As testing ramped up vigorously in April, the highest single "daily new cases" addition was April 24, at 38,958.[227] A "case" is a positive test where someone has SARS-CoV-2 with no symptoms, tests for antibodies for it, or has COVID-19.[228]

A person who had contracted SARS-CoV-2 and showed no symptoms might be immune and may have antibodies validating that. Someone who had COVID-19 and recovered would likely also have antibodies. A person developing immunity to a pathogen through infection typically takes place over 1-2 weeks.

Initially, with SARS-CoV-2 novel, there were not wide tests to see who had it. It was more like HIV early on. You'd get tested when you had some kind of symptoms that fit the associated diseases. Now, many people get tested for HIV as a routine STD test or if you're in an at-risk group. Early on, no one really knew how many had it. With SARS-CoV-2, there was no wide testing early on beyond situations like the cruise ships or what South Korea and Iceland executed.

To determine a disease's fatality, mathematical models are used. In a perfect information world, you would take the number of fatalities and divide that by all people who had contracted the virus, or cases, and you get a percentage, the infection fatality rate. The overall fatality rate is the number of fatalities divided by the population. Unfortunately, no good fatality rate data existed when COVID-19 first broke.

Some initial predictions were fatality rate estimates up to 7.9%, impossible even early on. The best data available was from the cruise ships, the Roosevelt and what was happening in other countries early on. Based only on that, informed analysts knew only the following segments were at high risk:

- Elderly with weakened immune systems
- People with respiratory or previously discussed underlying conditions, mostly elderly
- Obesity in younger (than 65) people

"Cases" began to be the torch that those against reopening the country would carry. By the end of April 2020, we knew many, many more people had contracted SARS-CoV-2 than was reported, based on small studies discussed below. By the end of April, the United States recorded more than one million cases. By the end of June we recorded 2.5MM cases.

Cases were increasing daily. That's bad, right? Except, while cases were increasing, hospitalizations were dropping, as were COVID-19 deaths. We were learning every day that passed that COVID-19 was less dangerous to the general populace than the day before. And still, the reopening's crawled.

For all of the government-mandated policies, here is maybe the best thing they could have done to really determine caseloads and possible herd immunity or herd exposure in May:

- Mandate random testing of 10,000 people in large cities like in Dallas, San Jose, Pittsburgh, Orlando and Denver across all age groups
- Mandate random testing of 3,000 people in medium cities like Tucson, Tulsa, Lexington, Syracuse and Richmond

Would this mandate be an invasion of citizen rights? Probably, but wasn't the entire lockdown an invasion of rights? We can argue it was for a state of emergency and for the greater good, and if so, so could this data pooling. Data like this would have been extremely valuable in determining what was happening around the country.

The case data we received was reactive. With hospitalizations down, we had far more tests available than volunteers. There was never a test shortage in May, just not enough people were sick to bother getting tested. We saw case increases in

June, largely because of two things: people going to the hospital for non-COVID-19 issues were tested, and as employees returned to work, many were required to be tested first. We did get small windows into what was happening early illustrated in studies below.

CHELSEA, MASSACHUSETTS

Chelsea is a city in the Boston area, directly across the Mystic River from Boston. Chelsea is a very densely populated area of Boston. It's a working-class community and a majority of the population are Hispanic. As an experiment, a random testing of 200 possible COVID-19-positive residents was conducted by the city in mid-April 2020. The results were released on April 17.

Of the 200 tested, 64 tested positive for antibodies linked to the coronavirus and without symptoms. This test and result received little national attention. It was small, but the nearly 30% result was a credible reason to believe the infection rate was much higher than ever thought. Similar results of the U.S. population would show more than a hundred million people had it and weren't affected.[229]

PRISONS

On April 21 and 23, 2020, the Trousdale Turner Correctional Center in Tennessee conducted a COVID-19 test of 3,697 inmates for the virus or antibodies linked to it. The results were 747 tested positive and 2,950 negative, a 20% positive rate in the prison. None were symptomatic for anything. This news would scarcely make national news headlines or be talked about.[230]

In Ohio, Marion Correctional Institution houses 2,500 prisoners, "many of them older with pre-existing health conditions. After testing 2,300 inmates for the coronavirus, they were shocked. Of the 2,028 who tested positive, close to 95% had no symptoms. As mass coronavirus testing expands in prisons, large numbers of inmates are showing no symptoms.

In four state prison systems — Arkansas, North Carolina, Ohio and Virginia — 96% of 3,277 inmates who tested positive for the coronavirus were asymptomatic, according to interviews with officials and records reviewed by *Reuters*. That's out of 4,693 tests that included results on symptoms."[231]

In Louisiana, the Department of Safety and Corrections tested inmates and 347 tested positive for COVID-19, 221 of them were symptomatic, the rest were not, and five died from it. All five had underlying conditions. Louisiana has more than 40,000 people imprisoned so the actual number of those infected had to be much higher. One out of every thousand people in Louisiana are imprisoned. In their women's prison, nearly every inmate tested positive and two-thirds had no symptoms.[232]

SANTA CLARA, CALIFORNIA

Stanford University researchers in Santa Clara, California, where we now believe the first COVID-19 death occurred, tested 3,300 people in April. They concluded that as much as 4.16% of the county's population, 81,000 people, may have coronavirus antibodies. None were symptomatic. If that run rate were extrapolated, it would be close to 100 times more people had been exposed with no effects than previously thought.

The test was not random like the Chelsea or Trousdale test. People volunteered and the results were not peer reviewed or scrutinized. However, it was consistent with the testing in Chelsea and Trousdale.[233]

The Stanford study was led by Dr. Jay Bhattacharya, a professor of medicine at Stanford University. His study suggests a fatality rate at 0.1% – 0.2%, which places it "somewhere between 'little worse than the flu' to 'twice as bad as the flu' in terms of case fatality rate," Bhattacharya says.

This is far less than fatality rates experts shared with us early on, in the range of 1% and 8%, depending on the country, with the global fatality rate being in the 3% range. Those fatality rates are more consistent with flu rates: about twice to three times worse. If we knew that, would we have shut down entire economies and societies around the world?

UNIVERSITY OF SOUTHERN CALIFORNIA STUDY

"Based on testing results from 863 adults, the research team estimates that approximately 4.1% of the county's adult population has an antibody to the virus. Adjusting this estimate for the statistical margin of error implies about 2.8% to 5.6% of the county's adult population has an antibody to the virus — which translates to approximately 221,000 to 442,000 adults in the county who have been infected.

That estimate is 28 to 55 times higher than the 7,994 confirmed cases of COVID-19 reported to the county at the time of the study in early April. The number of COVID-related deaths in the county has now surpassed 600."[234]

That number was a lower rate than the other tests indicated, and still suggests many more people have or have had the coronavirus with no symptoms.

NEW YORK CITY
New York state released on April 23 a study where 3,000 tests were conducted on shoppers at grocery stores and big box retailers (like Target or Walmart). The results were nearly 14% tested positive for coronavirus antibodies.[235] That suggests a run rate of 2.7MM New York state residents positive, 10 times more than the official number at the testing date. Critics suggested it's falsely high because those out and about are more likely to be positive than those staying home. It's also minimizing that most spread occurred at home. If those at home were infected and were staying home, the rate may be much higher.

MIAMI
On Friday, April 24, researchers at University of Miami released a study suggesting 6% of residents in Dade County have coronavirus antibodies, which represented 165,000 of Dade's nearly three million residents. Officially, the state of Florida reported a little more than 10,000 cases at this time. The UM researchers tested 1,400 people of a pool of volunteers. About half of the people who tested positive showed no symptoms the previous 10 to 14 days.[236]

NEW CASTLE, DELAWARE
New Castle, Delaware gets the most out-of-the-box coronavirus testing award. The testers sampled human waste raw sewage for the signs of the virus. They compared the "prevalence of genetic fragments from the virus in fecal matter against local population data and sewage flow rates – all in an effort to estimate how many people may have the virus."[237] Their study, released April 23, resulted in an estimation that more than 15,000 people, 3% of the population for the sewage area, had the virus by April 14. That would be 15 times the number of actual cases reported there.

U.S.S. ROOSEVELT
The U.S.S. Roosevelt expanded testing from what we discussed earlier to all 4,800 crew members. Some crew members who tested negative previously tested positive later, suggesting either they caught it later or their virus count was too low initially to show up on a test. The latest test results released on April 28 showed 955 crew members positive, about 20% of the total.[238]

On another ship, the U.S.S. Ronald Reagan in Japan, an undisclosed number of sailors tested positive for coronavirus. The sailors showed no symptoms.[239]

HOMELESS TEST

In Boston on around April 10, testers went to the Pine Street Inn homeless shelter in Boston's South End because there were a few cases there. They performed a sweeping test of 397 people there. Of those 397, 146 people tested positive. None of them were symptomatic. That's a 37% rate of spread.[240]

TYSON FOODS

Tyson Foods has a pork processing plant in Logansport, Indiana. On April 30, Tyson announced they were voluntarily closing for a few days to clean the plant and sort out what to do when 890 of 2200 employees tested positive for the coronavirus. None were ill or symptomatic.[241] The headline was reported as a shocking bad news result, while in reality it was one more example that the coronavirus was just not that dangerous to people not in vulnerable groups. The Tyson "outbreak" resulted in an extended stay-at-home order in the county. And still, hospitals were empty of COVID-19 and other patients.

IRAN

On May 1, 2020 *medRxiv* published a study based on antibody testing in Iran.[242] That study concluded that hundreds of thousands of Iranians in just the Guilan province likely had asymptomatic reactions to SARS-CoV-2 and were carrying antibodies. Project that out to the country of Iran based on that positive test rate and the fatality rate was about 0.29%. That's three people per thousand, about one to two more per thousand than the flu. On May 1, that news was not seen on any news channel. We saw challenges to reopening on many news channels because there was not enough testing getting done. Meanwhile, hospitals were still empty.

CHILDREN

In a German study released on April 20, a study traced an infected child to his contact with 172 people. Every person with whom he had contact tested negative, including his own siblings.[243]

In the whitepaper "Children are not COVID-19 super spreaders: time to go back to school," published in BMJ Journals, Doctors Alasdair Munro and Saul Faust, both UK researchers, studied children with respect to infection and infectious spread and reported the following:

- *"Children are primary spreaders of influenza within a household*
- *Children could be significantly less likely to become infected than adults*
- *Children were not likely to be the index case in households*
- *A case study of a cluster in the French Alps included a child with COVID-19 who failed to transmit it to any other person, despite exposure to more than a hundred children in different schools and a ski resort*
- *In New South Wales, Australia none of 735 students and 128 staff contracted COVID-19 from nine child and nine adult initial school cases despite close contact*
- *In the Netherlands, separate data from primary care and household studies suggests SARS-CoV-2 is mainly spread between adults and from adult family members to children*
- *There has been very little evidence so far on the effects of COVID-19 on children with comorbidities. This contrasts significantly to COVID-19 disease in adults.*
- *Governments worldwide should allow all children back to school regardless of comorbidities"*[244]

CHAPTER 17

REOPENING CRITERIA AND TESTING

By May 1, many states began reopening with many restrictions. In mid-April, the federal government had set guidelines of a 14-day decline in cases to reopen. Following that guideline would be inconsistent and then ignored by many states. The media pounced on that strategy, claiming it was "Russian roulette" to open without at least tens of millions more tests. The mainstream media criticized the Trump Administration for not getting enough tests complete, that we were missing targets. Somewhere along the month of April we lost our way.

This headline ran in *The New York Times* in April: *Testing Is Biggest Obstacle to Reopening States, Experts Say*.[245] Testing was available. The light testing didn't have anything to do with capacity. Few people wanted to get tested. They weren't symptomatic, and they weren't going in.

On May 1, at an average urgent care type of facility in New York City, the wait was less than a half hour to get in and out. In Los Angeles, Dallas, Detroit, same thing. In Dallas, the cost per test was $300 if you were not positive. Who would pay that if they weren't sick?

What we did know from the case studies in the previous chapter is that many more people had it than any official numbers. The number of cases was rising and hospitalizations were dropping, as were fatalities. That would result in scraping to get every COVID-19 case and death counted as possible. The goal post got moved and we lost our way on the real data that mattered.

COMPARING COUNTRIES

With data on "cases" unreliable, because in every country there were vastly more positive people than testing showed, the most objective data comparisons are deaths per capita. It's the closest reliable "scorecard" to evaluate the COVID-19 impact, and to evaluate the impact different measures had on decreasing deaths.

Case counts continued for weeks on the corners of cable news television screens. It was a meaningless number and would inject fear because in an absolute sense, without context, it's scary. A million people in America infected with the virus?! In reality, cases were going up by thousands a day while hospitalizations and deaths were decreasing, a great sign. That connection would scarcely be covered in major media outlets.

SWEDEN

Sweden was a center of worldwide controversy during the COVID-19 pandemic. Along with Japan, Sweden's leadership opted not to impose lockdowns on their society or economy. People were free to work, shop, dine out, ski and most children went to school. Sweden's leadership did stress hand washing, social distancing and protecting people over the age of 70 by limiting contact with them and banning visits to elderly care facilities.

Most of the population voluntarily social distanced, something they were counting on through citizen empowerment to slow the spread of the virus. South Dakota's governor Kristi Noem, the smartest governor in the room, employed a similar strategy.

Usage of public transport dropped significantly, large numbers worked from home, and the government banned gatherings of more than 50 people.

The strategy was that some exposure to SARS-CoV-2 built immunity among the general population while insulating the elderly. It would prove to be a winning strategy in the big picture while the elderly in nursing homes would suffer a fate similar to other countries. It would also be one of the boldest moves in Sweden's history.

Sweden was widely criticized for this by media figures around the world. Incredibly, on April 29, 2020, the World Health Organization (WHO) commended Sweden's approach as a "model" for other countries. Dr. Mike Ryan, the WHO's top emergencies expert, said there are *"lessons to be learned" from the Scandinavian nation.* That same Dr. Ryan said this in mid-March: *"The danger right now with the lockdowns ... if we don't put in place the strong public health measures now, when those movement restrictions and lockdowns are lifted, the danger is the disease will jump back up.*" He communicated even lockdowns were not enough. Once the smoke cleared from the wildfire, not locking down was enough.

It's a lovely example of why every citizen should research issues and draw their own conclusions, not solely relying on "experts" or the government, particularly in times of crisis when decisions are made quickly. All of the "experts" in industry and government are still people, people with predispositions and biases in some cases, and not necessarily clear thinking at that.

When the pandemic first hit America in March, friends were telling me this could go on all year, the world would never be the same, apocalyptic predictions. I was studying the data and suggested back when Dallas first locked down (third week of March) that there was no way this was going on past May 1, the data never supported it. They thought I was crazy. On May 1, dozens of states were still holding out, and hopefully voters will remember those decisions at their next election.

JAPAN

Japan also chose not to lockdown, very similar to Sweden's approach. Japan declared a state of emergency on April 7, and prior to that, testing was done on a wide range of the population. In a study from *medRxiv* published on May 1, 2020, the paper stated that it is unrealistic to find every case of those who had contracted SARS-CoV-2. They smartly referred back to the Diamond Princess data in addition to their own findings.

Their conclusion was that an average of 600 times more people had contracted it than are identified. That brought the fatality rate in line with the flu. They concluded that Japan was infected similar to western countries, but they were inconclusive why the fatality rates were lower.[246] This report was not seen in the mainstream media news cycle on May 1.

Japan and Sweden did not lock down, and Germany had a lighter lockdown than peer EU countries. Other countries locked down included in the chart on the next page, some in a near-military approach as previously discussed. By the time the pandemic deaths were on the decline, how did they fare?

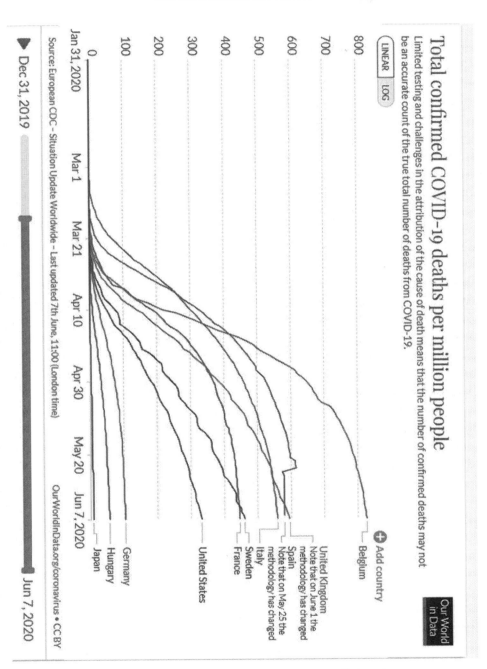

Total confirmed COVID-19 deaths per million people

Limited testing and challenges in the attribution of the cause of death means that the number of confirmed deaths may not be an accurate count of the true total number of deaths from COVID-19.

LINEAR LOG

800
700
600
500
400
300
200
100
0

Jan 31, 2020   Mar 1   Mar 21   Apr 10   Apr 30   May 20   Jun 7, 2020

Source: European CDC – Situation Update Worldwide – Last updated 7th June, 11:00 (London time)   OurWorldInData.org/coronavirus • CC BY

Dec 31, 2019   Jun 7, 2020

⊕ Add country

Belgium
United Kingdom
Note that on June 1 the methodology has changed
Spain
Note that on May 25 the methodology has changed
Italy
Sweden
France
United States
Germany
Hungary
Japan

Our World in Data

Comparing countries per capita deaths, per million. Source: https://ourworldindata.org/coronavirus-data?country=USA+HUN+ITA+JPN+ESP+SWE+GBR+FRA+DEU

199

Japan, which did not lockdown, is barely measurable on the chart over the page. They had no statistically significant COVID-19 fatalities. Germany, which locked down "light," was also very low. The United States fared with fewer than average fatalities. If you extract New York City out of the data, the United States would be around the Germany/Hungary level. However, New York City, if its own country, was highest. We've discussed the integrity of that data, but no matter the numbers, New York faced a crisis no one else in America had witnessed, and in no way is this analysis discounting that.

Sweden, which did not lock down at all came in average. Not surprising, the two European countries hit the hardest, Italy and Spain, are the highest. Recall that Belgium counted COVID-19 deaths different than other countries.

U.S. COMPARISONS

Let's compare South Dakota, a state that did not lockdown but did protect their elderly, to neighboring Idaho, which had much tighter restrictions during the lock-downs. Both are predominately rural states, lightly populated per square mile. Both were underwhelmed. Idaho has about 1.75MM residents and South Dakota has about 780,000. Below is their COVID-19 death rate per capita. Both are very low, but South Dakota had fewer COVID-19 fatalities. Statistically both were the same.

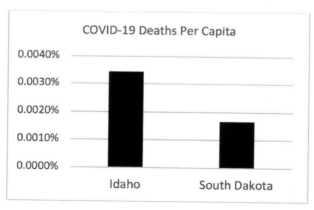

Source: https://www.worldometers.info/coronavirus/country/us/

Iowa had much lighter restrictions during the lockdown than neighboring Kansas. Iowa has 3.2MM residents and Kansas has 2.9MM residents. Below is their COVID-19 death rate per capita. Iowa is higher, and in absolute data Iowa had twenty-one more COVID-19 deaths with 300,000 more residents than Kansas for the same period through the end of April. Statistically both were the same.

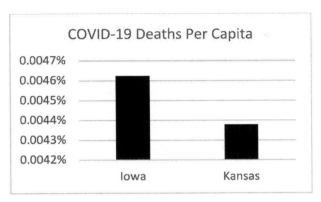

Source: https://www.worldometers.info/coronavirus/country/us/

So, did lockdowns matter? We'll never know, we can just debate it. The curves were set in motion before the lockdowns occurred anywhere. We never reached any of the early model predictions of hospitalizations or deaths. U.S. all-cause mortality is about even to previous years. Each country chose different paths to address it. The ones that did nothing or very little had no greater impact than those that did. In Japan's case, it scored best in the world.

States that had the lightest lockdowns were no worse impacted than those that had harsher lockdowns. What this data does illuminate is that it's unlikely the lockdowns had an impact worthy of the social and economic impacts it caused in the United States.

With the data known by May 1, we knew that the only people at risk were the elderly and those with specific pre-existing conditions. A very narrow and identifiable segment. Still, political leaders took what felt like forever to allow citizens to return to normal.

It became a pitching exercise and bad baseball management. If you fear a lineup when facing a team, you manage that. You can't walk the whole team to avoid them hitting because you will lose. Look at all-time leaders in walks. It's a Hall of Fame list. Why walk them? Because those batters could be isolated as the most dangerous and therefore pitchers would opt to avoid letting them hit, but pitch to the others. They identified risk, avoided it, and got on with the rest of the game. Sadly, our leaders chose to walk everyone, and we lost big when it was all over.

KEY TAKEAWAYS:

- Total deaths in the United States as the re-openings were debated were flat to the previous three-year average
- The New York City area was unusually affected in all-cause deaths more than anywhere in America
- More than half of the COVID-19 deaths occurred in nursing homes and this was not pre-empted with preventive policies early on
- The median age of all victims exceeded life expectancy in all countries
- There was no measurable risk to anyone under 65 without the underlying conditions discussed
- There was no measurable or identifiable risk of spread outdoors

FACE MASKS

In June 2020 wearing face masks became required or encouraged nearly everywhere. Is that helpful? According to an analysis[247] in *The Lancet*, wearing a non-respirator face covering (N95s are respirators) is not useful in stopping pathogens or airborne particles: "Surgical masks and cloth masks do not offer protection from inhaling particles or pathogens in the air—for that, you need to turn to respirators."

In addition to that, even if you wear one, to be effective, the fit around your nose and facial features is critical. So when you hear politicians or businesses telling us that we must wear "face coverings" in public, with no qualifier that a respirator-type is necessary for the protection of SARS-CoV-2, know they likely know nothing about what they're talking about.

SOCIAL DISTANCING

Social distancing became the worldwide practice and buzzword in the spring of 2020. According to the CDC:

> "Social distancing, also called 'physical distancing,' means keeping space between yourself and other people outside of your home. To practice social or physical distancing:

- *Stay at least 6 feet (about 2 arms' length) from other people*
- *Do not gather in groups*
- *Stay out of crowded places and avoid mass gatherings"*

In early May, I went to the Walmart Neighborhood Market; the parking lot was fairly open as usual. When I got to the checkout, there were lines three to four people deep, this was unusual based on the number of cars in the parking lot. When I got to the self-checkout line, I then saw every other checkout was closed, and a sign was on the closed ones reading "This checkout is closed to maintain social distancing of six feet."

Meanwhile, all the shoppers were equally handling produce, boxed goods, touching the checkout screens and point of sale. It was an absurd inconsistency and really demonstrating that there was no need to close the other checkout lanes.

My neighborhood has many parks nearby, and one has a five-foot-wide 100-foot bridge over a creek. Even during the lockdown, the parks were pretty active with people enjoying spring outdoors. A woman posted on our Nextdoor app that people should wait at one end of the bridge or the other if someone was already on the bridge to practice social distancing. She then vented about kids hanging together at the shore of a small lake nearby. Sentiments like this were felt all over the country, just go back and read social media comments from March through June of 2020.

The Lancet published an analysis[248] on June 1 2020 with medium to low certainty that social distancing of one meter helps curb the spread and two meters does a little better. They also found that wearing medical grade face masks helped curb infection spread by the wearer, and that medical grade (N95-type) are better than cotton ones commonly used. The study also stated "At present, there is no data to support viable virus in the air outside of aerosol generating procedures from available hospital studies." Which means, wearing a mask in the outdoors or your car or where you are not in close contact with others is meaningless.

CNN reported this in April 2020: "U.S. may have to endure social distancing until 2022 if no vaccine is quickly found, scientists predict."[249] It was an absurd suggestion. The reason countries were locked down was to flatten the hospitalization curve. This never happened anywhere in America beyond the New York area and a few hospitals in Detroit and New Orleans, and all of those for only two to three weeks and none of those cities reached actual capacity.

By late April 2020, "the only thing flatter than the hospitalization curve was the economy" (quote credit to Alex Berenson). SARS-CoV-2 spread most commonly within households, nursing homes, then through hospitals and to a much lower degree, public transportation.

The quickest way to get through this, assuming that in the absence of a vaccine to achieve herd immunity, was to integrate. By the time the lockdowns were winding down in May 2020, data was everywhere that the virus had spread much wider than anyone knew. A million cases were reported, but people in the know knew it had to be closer to a hundred million than one million.

We knew the fatality rate was very low, a little worse than the flu. A flu virus might kill one person in one to two thousand people who catch it. COVID-19 is higher, maybe 2-3 people in one to two thousand. We knew the vulnerable segments of the population. We knew children and healthy adults were at no measurable risk.

What was the hold-up? Why were citizens and leadership in local, states and the federal government reluctant to encourage everyone getting back to normal?

The media.

CHAPTER 18

DIRTY LAUNDRY

Sitting in English class one day as a high school junior, my teacher Mr. Miller, the best teacher I ever had, called on me in a Socratic tone and asked me to explain to the class the meaning of the current hit, "Dirty Laundry." At the time I was the most knowledgeable student in the school about pop music history, never getting to apply that on a game show quiz. That year, I wrote a 20-page paper on John Lennon's influence on American pop culture in a couple of days, all from memory. The hard work was in finding the bibliography sources for all of this useless information.

I didn't know the lyrics to "Dirty Laundry," and my classmate Vicki stepped up and filled us all in. The Don Henley hit speaks of the thirst for the cutting storyline in the media, the zest for bad news and the desire to get the headline ignoring facts sometimes. At the time, I was too young to really get it. Even as I got older, I thought media bias was more a commentary from a disgruntled subject. But a little later it jumped out.

There are different kinds of media bias. One form is the omission of facts. You can provide some information but not all, just sharing the data that supports the "journalist" point of view. "Journalist" is in quotations because there are so few. If an actual journalist, the person has an obligation to facts, reporting accurate information to the reader or listener. That must be a little boring because there are so few high-profile ones out there.

Another kind of media bias is simply choosing what to report on. This is most prevalent today. Watch the network and cable news one day nonstop, flipping channels between ABC/CBS/NBC nightly news, and cable news on CNN, Fox News, MSNBC and One America News. Most days you will see different topics covered on the same news day. Nearly all cable news is opinion reporting, with few reporting objectively on the day's events. No news show is opinion-free on MSNBC or CNN. There isn't anything wrong with that, it can be great entertainment, particularly if it supports your point of view. It's just not journalism.

CABLE AND ONLINE NEWS

Fox News has been the highest-rated cable news network for decades. MSNBC has been the second highest-rated cable news network and CNN third. Political coverage is liberal-leaning on MSNBC and CNN, and conservative-leaning on Fox News and One America News. Here's a gauge as to whether a television news show is opinion-based or actual journalism: if a show is consistently criticizing one political party and never reporting on anything good, it's a good indicator it's an opinion show.

Vox, Slate and *Daily Beast*, among others, write analysis or opinions from a liberal point of view. *Breitbart, Townhall, The Washington Examiner* and others do the same thing from a conservative perspective. News is usually created and read to support an existing political or social view, not to create a new one. Everyone should absorb points of view from both sides on everything and checking more than one source on major issues.

SOCIAL MEDIA

Social media is a bigger news influencer today than anything you see on cable news or in major news outlets like *The New York Times* or *The Washington Post*. Some 326 million people live in America. Fox News gets 3.5 million viewers on their best day, CNN never reaching a million and MSNBC between the two. A half million people read *The New York Times* daily and twice that on Sundays. That's with eight million people alone in New York City.

It's crazy how some people get so wrapped up in Fox News's conservative perspective when they only reach 1% of America on their best day, and it's likely the same all the time. It's a small sliver of Americans that watch cable news and those viewers are 1% mostly solidified in their political and social beliefs.

Social media is another story. It's shaping the news, what people see, read, believe. With attention spans shorter than ever, getting quick news bites from Twitter and Facebook is much more impacting than deeper-dive opinion shows and opinion editorials. Twitter has 48 million users in America. Facebook has more than 200 million users.

Around 34% of Americans polled said they prefer to get their news from online media.[250] Four of 10 Americans prefer to get their news from Facebook. Compare that to one in 300 get their news from Fox News. Around 57% of those viewers said they believe the news they see online is inaccurate.

Unfortunately, social media companies censored even reasoned data or contrarian opinion that challenged the COVID-19 shutdowns. When two California doctors who run urgent care centers challenged the need for California's shutdown, based on what they see at their clinics, YouTube removed their statements. YouTube stated the platform's policy is to ban content that "disputes the efficacy of health authority recommended guidance." Reminder: these "authorities" thought banning flights from China in January was a bad idea and that all ages were affected equally from the coronavirus in March.

Free speech? Who is YouTube to be the arbiter of what quality guidance is? If this pandemic proved anything, "experts" are people like you and me and often predisposed, meaning, they're human. Those predispositions often come before objective analysis. If a health expert still recommended lockdowns in June as a good idea and questioned schools opening in the fall (see Dr. Fauci), their laptop should be taken away and they should be sent to their rooms without WiFi to connect them to the outside world.

Twitter began censoring and removing any tweets and information they deemed as disputing COVID-19 information.[251] Twitter techs became the arbiters of accurate medical information. It wouldn't matter that much of the information from "official" sources was misleading in itself. Now one of the largest media companies in the world was censoring information. Who could blame most people from being scared when they were insulated from data and varying points of view? Not one media outlet reported the United States was actually down at the beginning of May in all-cause deaths compared to expectations, by thousands. If it were even within 2-3% of normal, it should have been headline news.

Facebook shut down the page for Michiganders Against Excessive Quarantine (385,000 members) in May 2020, the group organizing protests in Michigan. They started up a new page called Stand Up Michigan, another protest group page, and it was shut down immediately, while a page called Stand Up America that was critical of the Trump administration was still up.

The media shaped the COVID-19 story, and that drove polls in an election year that drove politicians to shut down states and keep the social and economic fabric down into the greatest freefall in American history.

APPROVAL RATINGS IN THE SPRING 2020[252]

- President Trump, April 24, 2020--   44% Approval
- Congress, April 2020--   29% Approval
- Right Direction of the Country--   35% Approval

AMERICA'S HANDLING OF THE COVID-19 CRISIS, MARCH 2020:

	APPROVE	DISAPPROVE
Your hospital	88%	10%
Your state government	82%	17%
Government Health Agencies	80%	17%
President Trump	60%	38%
Congress	59%	37%
The Media	44%	55%

Source: Gallup, https://news.gallup.com/poll/300680/coronavirus-response-hospitals-rated-best-news-media-worst.aspx

Gallup released the poll results below in September 2019. Over the past 20years, there was a gradual decline in media trust. The poll reached an all-time low during the 2016 election, no doubt the polarizing election coverage drove that to a lower approval rating of either candidate or party. There's an irony when the media polls lower than a candidate, or when Congress polls lower than the president. Within that poll, respondents said they trust the media to varying degrees, and just 13% have a great deal of trust in the media:

- 13% have a great deal of trust
- 28% a fair amount
- 30% not very much
- 28% none at all

AMERICANS' TRUST IN MASS MEDIA	
1999	55%
2004	44%
2005	50%
2008	43%
2011	42%
2013	44%
2016	32%
2017	41%
2019	41%

Source: https://news.gallup.com/poll/267047/americans-trust-mass-media-edges-down.aspx

INITIAL MEDIA COVERAGE

The media shaped the COVID-19 story and played a critical role in the lock-downs, the re-openings, and who's to blame for the crisis. Back in January and February 2020, the media downplayed the pandemic. No one really saw this coming and impacting like it did, both in health impacts and the state-by-state closings. Below are some headlines that ran in major publications early on:

- *Worried About Catching The New Coronavirus? In The U.S., Flu Is A Bigger Threat*[253]
- *Something far deadlier than the Wuhan coronavirus lurks near you, right here in America. The virus is influenza, and it poses a far greater threat to Americans than the coronavirus from China that has made headlines around the world.*[254]
- *Coronavirus is spreading — but the flu is a greater threat to Americans*[255]
- *Get a grip, America. The flu is a much bigger threat than coronavirus, for now.*[256]

On January 30, 2020, CNN's Alisyn Camerota and Dr. Sanjay Gupta discussed on-air that the season's flu was a much bigger threat than SARS-CoV-2. On March 1, on NBC *Nightly News*, the anchor said with a graphic depicting one COVID-19 death to 12,000-60,000 flu deaths already in 2020. On January 22, Dr. John Torres was on NBC News saying that while a lot of people were talking about the coronavirus, the real threat to Americans was the flu.

On January 25, the *Good Morning America* team discussed the coronavirus and said it was a reminder to look out for the flu that season. On January 27, Dr. Dave Campbell spoke on MSNBC's *Morning Joe* and advised that the virus panic in China was a wakeup call for Americans to pay attention to the flu that winter. Another CNN report on February 1, stated the flu was a much bigger threat to America than the coronavirus. Dr. David Argus spoke on CBS *This Morning* on February 8 and said that the coronavirus was not going to cause a major issue in the United States.

The point of revisiting these comments is not to indict these people for poor reporting, it wasn't. It's to demonstrate that early on, no one saw the pandemic impacting the United States in any meaningful way. No one except Steve Bannon. Bannon's War Room show shifted in early January to *War Room: Pandemic*. Bannon, the smartest guy in any room at any time, identified the pandemic's impact on the world well before any other analyst or media figure. If you think that's biased, even Bill Maher lavished such praise on Bannon, telling him during an interview on his show in September 2018 that he "wished he worked for the other side."

CHINA TRAVEL HALTED

On January 31, President Trump halted flights and incoming travelers not American from entering the United States. Here are some of the reaction to that decision:

> *Health experts warn China travel ban will hinder coronavirus response*[257]

Former Vice President Joe Biden and presidential candidate:

> *"We have, right now, a crisis with the coronavirus. This is no time for Donald Trump's record of hysteria and xenophobia - hysterical xenophobia - and fearmongering to lead the way instead of science."*[258]

We saw Mr. Biden very critical of President Trump's slow-to-move actions to impede the virus spreading within the United States. On May 5, Mr. Biden said *"President Trump will try to paper over his administration's failed response to the COVID-19 pandemic when he travels today to Arizona — but nothing can cover up how he failed to prepare our country for this pandemic and his slow response."*[259]

If Mr. Biden is correct, it would be helpful to explain exactly how and to put some math behind his reasoning. For all the generalities politicians and pundits would use in their criticism, hopefully one journalist will ask a few questions deep enough to explain exactly how.

World Health Organization Chief Tedros Adhanom Ghebreyesus said on February 3, there was no need for measures that *"unnecessarily interfere with international travel and trade"* in trying to halt the spread of a coronavirus that has killed 361 people in China.[260]

On cable news, there were echoes of criticism for the move. In February, discussions of the coronavirus were mounting in the United States. Still, no one really thought it was going to impact us and no one imagined the United States doing a Wuhan-like lockdown here at home.

In early February, Dr. Anthony Fauci said, *"It's very, very transmissible, and it almost certainly is going to be a pandemic, but will it be catastrophic? I don't know."* That *The New York Times* article went on to say *"Closing borders to highly infectious pathogens never succeeds completely, experts said, because all frontiers are somewhat porous. Nonetheless, closings and rigorous screening may slow the spread, which will buy time for the development of drug treatments and vaccines."*

On February 29, Dr. Fauci spoke on NBC's *Today Show* and explained how community spread works, but that at that time there was no need to change any lifestyle habits. That tone changed in just two weeks.

EUROPEAN FLIGHTS HALTED

As things heated up in America and in Europe, President Trump then halted flights between European nations and the United States. Reaction to that drew criticism:

Public Health Experts Question Trump's Ban On Most Travelers From Europe: "From a public health perspective, it's remarkably pointless," says Francois Balloux, an epidemiologist at University College London who worked with the World Health Organization on the 2009 H1N1 flu pandemic. Balloux says closing borders only works in the very early days of an outbreak, or for countries that haven't yet detected any cases at all.[261]

Other political reaction from Europe was equally critical: Charles Michel, president of the European Council, and Ursula von der Leyen, president of the European Commission, issued a joint statement, saying, "The European Union disapproves of the fact that the U.S. decision to

*impose a travel ban was taken unilaterally and without consultation."
The two EU representatives continued, "The coronavirus is a global crisis,
not limited to any continent, and it requires cooperation rather than
unilateral action."*

EU condemns Trump travel ban from Europe as virus spreads[262]

*"Trump needed a narrative to exonerate his administration from any
responsibility in the crisis," Gérard Araud, the former French ambassador to
the U.S., tweeted on Wednesday. "The foreigner is always a good scapegoat.
The Chinese has already been used. So, let's take the European, not any
European, the EU-one. Doesn't make sense but ideologically healthy."*[263]

*Chaos in Europe, and Anger, Over U.S. Travel Ban to Curb Coronavirus;
European leaders denounced President Trump's decision to block most
visitors from the Continent for 30 days.*[264]

Former Vice President and presidential nominee Joe Biden took to Twitter
when this happened and wrote: *"A wall will not stop the coronavirus. Banning all
travel from Europe — or any other part of the world — will not stop it."* This same
nominee would repeatedly criticize President Trump for not doing enough early
on to stave off the spread.

Were the tables turned and a Democrat was leading the White House, there is
little doubt moves like this would have drawn fire from a high-profile Republican or
two and some in conservative media. Behind closed doors, would Mr. Biden have
criticized President Trump's travel bans to/from China and Europe? Doubtful.

Without a media microphone and an election year, the temperaments are
much milder behind the scenes. A thirsty media seeking a next high "Breaking
News!" headline, the media and viewers get addicted to dirty laundry.

The cost is journalism. It's so much more credible to criticize by giving some
recognition for something good or occasionally so one at least appears balanced
and then the criticism carries more weight [see Dana Perino].

COVID-19 REACHES AMERICA

The federal government's role in curtailing the pandemic early was to stop the spread from international infiltration, declare a national emergency, and ensure resources were available for states. The federal government did that. From there, states and governors had the authority to make their own guidelines tailored for their states. The situation in New York was vastly different than that in Iowa, for example.

What became very troubling is when finger-pointing began at two faces of the pandemic in America, President Trump and Mayor Bill de Blasio. Both were accused of "having blood on their hands" by their political opponents, the ugliest moment of politics in the pandemic.

Mayor de Blasio was reluctant to close schools in New York early on. First, concede it's much easier to sit on the couch and berate a coach or quarterback for calling or making a bad play. Imagine being faced with decisions of this potentially life and death, and economic, magnitude. Decisions the president, governors and city leaders like de Blasio made were the biggest policy decisions of their lives.

Here is some of the backlash de Blasio faced in the media:

'Blood on their hands:' Teachers say de Blasio and Carranza helped spread coronavirus[265]

Teachers Blame De Blasio, Schools Chancellor For Spread Of Coronavirus: 'The Blood Is on Their Hands'[266]

Mayor de Blasio was scolded in the media for also encouraging New Yorkers to get out and about in the city and not be afraid of the virus, very early on. That proved to be advice against the grain. In that moment, no one even then saw the sweeping crisis that overtook New York for the next three weeks. Regardless, anyone who thinks Mayor de Blasio has "blood on his hands" is reckless and mean-spirited and doesn't understand the data.

Whatever was going to happen in New York, the wheels were in motion before the lockdown. In hindsight, closing schools is a questionable decision. Academics suffered as discussed later, and no healthy children were at risk nor transmitters. We actually knew much of that from early analysis in March, but that data got shelved as panic set in.

President Trump faced similar media and political feedback. Political and media opponents repeated for months that the president acted too slow, that he, too, had blood on his hands:

March 29, 2020: "NBC's Chuck Todd under fire for asking Biden if Trump has 'blood on his hands' for delayed coronavirus response."[267] Mr. Biden fortunately did not take the bait, and said he thought that was a little too harsh. Still, when you consider how tight this time frame was, and the criticism the president took for halting travel between the United States and later Europe, and then declaring a national emergency, what exactly did critics want the federal government to do?

On March 17 (March 17!), Mike Broihier, a farmer and retired Marine, said in a video post "Because of Mitch, more people will die, more Kentuckians will die. Mitch has blood on his hands." How exactly would more Kentuckians die because of Mitch McConnell?[268]

On March 30, the Boston Globe editorial board accused the president of having "blood on his hands."[269] Politicians and pundits made these assertions and no responsible journalists seemed to ask exactly how they have blood on their hands, what exactly should have been done tactically, and what outcome would have been different and why.

On March 29, Speaker of the House Nancy Pelosi said, "Well, first of all, let me just say how sad it is that, even since the president's signing of the [coronavirus emergency bill], the number of deaths reported has doubled from 1,000 to 2,000 in our country. This is such a very, very sad time for us. So we should be taking every precaution. What the president — his denial at the beginning was deadly. His delaying of getting equipment to where — it continues — his delay in getting equipment to where it's needed is deadly."[270]

The problem with that is the equipment was everywhere it was needed. We fortunately never needed the navy ship docked in New York harbor, nor any extra ventilators that were such a hot topic for a couple of weeks. Interviewers never pressed any critics for any details.

In late February, Speaker Pelosi was out and about in San Francisco, dining in Chinatown. She commented that the city of San Francisco was on top of everything and encouraged others to get out. She was there to support the Chinese community amidst the controversy of the virus originating in China. What Pelosi did was fine, and she was really doing in late February a version of what de Blasio did in mid-March. It's not fair to criticize them for that at the time with what we knew, nor is it fair to criticize the president for inaction.

The reason for the grandstanding is the media. The press is a necessary check on reporting on the government. When is enough enough though? The politicians would never bother doing this if their words weren't printed or aired. Reflect back to how the country came together after the September 11 attacks. If that were an election year, would President Bush's opponents have leveraged that to blame him? We'll never know.

Politics began to get ugly after the close 2000 presidential election. It stepped up over the Iraq War, though support for that was definitely bipartisan. When President Obama was elected, it notched up more, largely because there were passionate adversaries to the Affordable Care Act, which passed completely along party lines. When President Trump ran and took office, with his open communication style and aggressive talk to his critics, politics became an MMA sport.

IN THE MIDST OF CHAOS

Into May 2020, a few things became clear:

- The New York City area was hit very hard and was on edge. While they never exceeded hospital capacity, it was a scary time for a few weeks.
- Other than Detroit and New Orleans for a couple of weeks, no other city or state had a high number of hospitalizations or deaths that were predicted.
- More than half of the deaths occurred within or sourced from nursing homes, maybe well over half when the counting is done.
- Almost no one under 65 was in a perilous situation unless they had then-known preexisting conditions, as discussed; 90%-plus of the COVID-19 deaths occurred in people with one or often more pre-existing conditions.
- Cases were rising while hospitalizations and fatalities were declining.
- Children were not affected.
- 40 million people lost their jobs and it was going to be an economic collapse of epic proportions.

With very little COVID-19 impact in most states, several groups began rumblings of reopening the economy. In late March, President Trump floated the idea of reopening on Easter Sunday, April 12. Many across the country were excited, though polls showed the country was fearing the virus and a high majority thought it was too soon. That date was soon dismissed, as the second week of April saw COVID-19 deaths peak.

The third week of April saw a sharp decline in hospitalizations, the leading indicator of deaths by about 10 days. If hospitalizations were down, deaths would decline. One thing never reported on during the entire pandemic was hospitalizations compared to capacity or expectations. You didn't see anything reported on all-cause deaths compared to previous year.

If you know anything about President Trump, he considers the economy his personal scorecard for his job approval. Whether you like him or not, most of his policies and conversations are usually pointed toward economic policy. With the economy somewhere between on hold and in ruins, and with COVID-19 deaths not reaching the predicted apocalypse, he was visibly itching to reopen states and get people back to work.

POLLING

In an April 15, 2020 poll by NBC and the Wall Street Journal, 45% of the respondents said the country should reopen in the next few weeks, 26% in the next year and 6% longer than a year.[271] Pew Research released a poll on April 16. In that, 65% of the respondents said the president acted too slow in preparing America for the virus, 66% felt the states would reopen too quickly, and 73% felt the worst was yet to come.[272] With hospitalizations on the decline, only 2-3 pockets hit hard and now declining and 40 million Americans out of work, why was America so scared? The media coverage.

In looking at objective data, when America was locked down, there was initial fear that 2.2MM people would lose their lives. That went down to 150,000-200,000 within 10 days, and then it went down to a range of 60,000-150,000. Given that as the benchmark for what America was expecting, how were we faring?

To compare, we need to look at different countries and their COVID-19 deaths per million, revisiting an earlier chart. The United States would naturally be a leader in total pandemic deaths because it's so large, and the data from China was unreliable. As of May 4, every country was on the decline. Below are the total deaths per million for select countries, a key date because this was at the height of debates to reopen states.[273] Recall that Japan and Sweden did not lock down at all and Germany locked down light.

COUNTRY	COVID-19 DEATHS PER MILLION, MAY 4, 2020	COVID-19 DEATHS PER MILLION, JUNE 17, 2020[1]
Spain	540	580
Italy	478	570
United Kingdom	419	623
France	381	453
Sweden	265	500
United States	204	362
Canada	98	219
Germany	80	107
Iran	74	110
South Korea	5	5
Japan	4	7

Source: https://www.worldometers.info/coronavirus/#countries

If you considered the New York City metro area (including parts of New Jersey and Connecticut) its own country for this exercise, the death rate would be more than a thousand per million, by far the largest proportionate hit in the world. And, if you took that same area out of the rest of the United States, the deaths per million would be around 250 in June.

By any measure, it's illogical to suggest anyone acted slow, thus resulting in thousands of deaths that would not have happened. In total, the United States fared better than France, Spain, Italy, the United Kingdom, and Sweden. If we were first expecting more than two million deaths, then 150,000, and we came in well below that, isn't that some degree of success? If you believed that COVID-19 was as deadly as the media had us believe, then you'd have to feel the United States survived well.

My belief is, having studied all this data in the United States and Europe, had we done nothing, we would have ended up within 20% of where we were with the lockdowns by mid-May and exactly where we ended up by August. It is likely that like other respiratory viruses, we will see a future cold-air spike. Had we done nothing but quarantined nursing homes and long-term-care facilities, not allowed any positive-testing people to work, visit or reside there, we would've done better than having locked everyone down. We did not act surgically, and the data was there early on to have done so.

Below are select states' COVID-19 deaths per million as the reopening debate was in full force:

	COVID-19 DEATHS PER MILLION ON MAY 4, 2020
New York	1,271
New Jersey	895
Connecticut	714
Massachusetts	599
Michigan	415
Illinois	208
Georgia	121
Washington	116
Florida	68
California	58
Texas	33
Oregon	27
South Dakota	24

We never saw this data broadcast in major print media articles nor on network or cable news. For some context, 800 people per day lose their lives in Texas, 1,000 per day in California. This was very grounding data that suggested while this was no flu virus, the type and number of deaths were much closer to a bad flu season than a pandemic worthy of:

- 40 million people losing their jobs
- Trillions of dollars of government bailouts
- Social dysfunction
- Non-covid-19 health implications of medical treatments delayed and the lasting effect that may have

MOVING THE GOAL POST

In mid-to-late April, the media moved the goal posts. Hospitalization tallies were never discussed in the media, that capacity was never reached and most hospitals were as empty as the closed trails in Yosemite National Park. On March 28, when President Trump suggested reopening on Easter, a report was published called "National Coronavirus Response: A Road Map to Reopening." It was released by The American Enterprise Institute in collaboration with faculty from the Johns Hopkins Center for Health Security.

Crystal Watson and Caitlin Rivers authored the report, both senior scholars at the Center for Health Security.[274] In their report, they recommended the following, per an interview with Watson:

- *"For a phase one reopening, no state relax physical distancing until it sees a sustained reduction in cases for at least 14 days, its hospitals can safely treat all patients without resorting to crisis standards of care, and it's able both to test all people with COVID-19 symptoms, and conduct monitoring of confirmed cases and their contacts.*

- *We need to build capacity at hospitals—beds, ventilators, protective equipment—and create facilities for people with the illness to recover in isolation if they are unable to stay at home.*

- *In Phase II, schools, universities, and businesses may begin to reopen (albeit in a modified way to reduce opportunity for transmission)—but teleworking should continue where convenient, and social gatherings should continue to be limited to fewer than 50 people wherever possible. Opening schools is a tough one because having kids in school, as we've seen with flu, could be a driver of infection."*

Into late-April, COVID-19 hospitalizations were on a steep decline, even in New York and Detroit. In Watson's defense at the time her report was authored, a lot of new data came to light in just three weeks. What got lost is that the reason we locked down in the first place was to avoid overwhelming hospitals to where sick COVID-19 patients could not receive care. With that no longer at risk, what was the delay in reopening? The mood in mid-to-late April shifted to politics.

The media was pounding the case increases every day, and deaths were still increasing, but less and less per day. Real deaths and back-dated deaths, they were certainly growing, but not to any model degree and not justifying the social and economic lockdowns.

Each day on cable news, on the right side of the screen in red boxes they displayed the number of cases in America and the number of deaths. In absolute numbers it looked scary. In the context of what was not just really happening but what happens every year in America, it was not. Cases became the new mantra in news reporting. Cases was viewed as a bad thing. However, it was not.

Cases grew as hospitalizations and deaths dropped, and any sixth-grade math student could identify an inverse relationship happening. If cases were growing and hospitalizations and deaths were growing commensurately, that would be a trend worthy of continuing measures or doing something different. They weren't.

On May 4, the United States saw the lowest daily death total for a single day in more than a month. That became a headline on exactly one news source, at 10 p.m. on the evening of May 5 on *Breitbart*. We reached a three-month low of COVID-19 deaths in June, also not covered in the news.

TAKING SIDES

As the country began to debate reopening, liberal media figures were adamantly opposed to it, while conservative media was all about reopening. It became completely political. Was this because of the upcoming election? The economy was President Trump's greatest accomplishment to promote. Would Democrat-led states and liberal media really believe COVID-19 was still a broad-sweeping threat worthy of shutting down schools and the economy, the social fabric of America? I asked everyone I knew if they thought the media and political leaders opposed to reopening was out of genuine fear of the virus or to keep the economy down to hurt President Trump's reelection chances. This isn't a conspiracy theory, because the sides of reopening versus remaining locked down were closely tied to party lines by now.

THE NEW YORK TIMES

Tom Friedman is a writer for *The New York Times*. In 1989, Friedman wrote a very comprehensive and terrific book called *From Beirut to Jerusalem*. I read it in the moment as a college student and loved it, you should check it out even now. While

Friedman was no supporter of President George W. Bush, he did write of reasons to justify the Iraq War.[275] It was disappointing to see. While the Iraq War was debated and beginning, my dad and I sat around watching the news shaking our heads at that decision – how on earth was Iraq a threat to American interests, with zero proof they were involved in the September 11 attacks?

Friedman has nothing but disdain for President Trump. As an opinion writer that's fine, healthy and fair to offer his point of view. During the discussions of reopening the country, the opinion writer made some reckless commentary about the president and the associated risks of reopening. In an April 18, 2020 column in *The New York Times*, the headline read "*Trump Is Asking Us to Play Russian Roulette With Our Lives.*"[276] In the piece, Friedman wrote:

- *"'LIBERATE MINNESOTA!' 'LIBERATE MICHIGAN!' "LIBERATE VIRGINIA.' With these three short tweets last week, President Trump attempted to kick off the post-lockdown phase of America's coronavirus crisis. It should be called: 'American Russian roulette: The Covid-19 version." What Trump was saying with those tweets was: Everybody just go back to work. From now on, each of us individually, and our society collectively, is going to play Russian roulette. We're going to bet that we can spin through our daily lives — work, shopping, school, travel — without the coronavirus landing on us. And if it does, we'll also bet that it won't kill us.*

- *More specifically: As a society, we will be betting that as large numbers of people stop sheltering in place, the number of people who will still get infected with Covid-19 and require hospitalization will be less than the number of hospital beds, intensive care units, respirators, doctors, nurses and protective gear needed to take care of them.*

- *Because it is clear that millions of Americans are going to stop sheltering in place — their own President is now urging them to liberate themselves — before we have a proper testing, tracking and tracing system set up. Until we have a vaccine, that kind of system is the only path to dramatically lowering the risk of infection while partially opening society — while also protecting the elderly and infirm — as Germany has demonstrated.*

- *'Liberate?' Think about the use of that word. We were not in jail! We were not doing something wrong! We were doing what our president, governor, mayor, and national epidemic experts told us to do: behave responsibly and shelter in place to break the transmission of this virus."*

The flaws in Friedman's argument are numerous. Russian roulette, strictly speaking, is when you load one bullet in a revolver, spin the chamber, and pull the trigger, with a fully equal one in six chance of dying. There is a haunting scene depicting this in the classic film, *The Deer Hunter*. Russian roulette gives everyone an equal probability of dying.

COVID-19 did not give everyone an equal probability of getting sick much less dying. Only clearly identified segments of the population were at risk, and that was who needed insulation and protection. With the economy on fire, hospitalizations and deaths declining, and knowing who was at risk, requiring vast testing and tracing was not a reasonable requirement to opening the country up. Washington Governor Jay Inslee required just that (on May 18, 2020) to open up Washington.

Friedman is a smart man and accomplished journalist. Did he actually believe what he wrote, or was his dislike for President Trump motivating this? Friedman's next article was titled, *"We Need Herd Immunity From Trump and the Coronavirus."* The one after that was, *"Is Sweden Doing It Right? The Swedes aren't battling the coronavirus with broad lockdowns."* Perhaps Friedman was coming around.

This isn't about picking on Friedman; he was speaking metaphorically about Russian roulette. Messages like his and what you see on the news are enormous influencers on social media, which drive public opinion. Public opinion, as we saw in the polls, was largely scared as states began reopening. When print, online and television media promote scary news like cases growing, without context, it shapes public opinion and polls.

If the polls said most of the public think states should remain closed, politicians would follow to some degree. It was an election year. When Georgia governor Brian Kemp was the first to announce a reopening in late April, President Trump denounced the move in his daily briefing, saying it was too soon. Did he really think it was too soon? No chance. But with the majority of Americans polling that we should not reopen yet, President Trump was unusually measured.

By late April, headlines should have been seen all over America that would read something like this:

- *Cases rising while hospitalizations and fatalities drop*
- *Nursing homes at biggest risk for COVID-19*
- *United States faring better than most countries battling COVID-19*
- *Children at no measurable risk to COVID-19*
- *California largely untouched by COVID-19*
- *COVID-19 spread mostly through families*

Would coverage have been different if President Obama were still in office, and President Obama wanted to get things reopened? It's very likely that Democrat-led states would follow that lead. Would Republican-led states have resisted? It seems unlikely that governors like Greg Abbott or Ron DeSantis would not have reopened given what we knew by late April.

On April 21, *The Washington Post* ran a column titled, "*Georgia leads the race to become America's No. 1 Death Destination.*" In it, writer Dana Milbank blasted Florida, South Carolina and mostly Georgia for their plans to reopen.[277] One of the blames was the lack of testing. He predicted the coronavirus would burn through the people of Georgia like a fireball after they reopened. Had he looked at the data? Milbank closed in his piece:

"You and a guest are invited to LIBERATE GEORGIA!

The Grand Reopening of the Petri State

Grand Marshal: President Trump

Dress: PPE optional.

As a promotion, Georgia could offer ventilators to the first 100 hotel guests to register (room service would offer supplementary oxygen at no cost to all others). Atlanta's own Coca-Cola would sponsor festivities, using the new slogan 'Share a Coke with Covid-19.' The Atlanta Symphony Orchestra would perform a new variation on Berlioz, 'The Damnation of Fauci.' Trump and Kemp would lead a packed house at Atlanta's State Farm Arena in burning their face masks the way feminists (apocryphally) burned bras and Vietnam War protesters actually burned draft cards."

Milbank must not have studied the actual petri dish: the cruise ships. Weeks after the reopening, on May 19, Georgia's COVID-19 hospitalizations were down 34% for the month. Georgia had lost 155 people per million to COVID-19 and had an overall fatality rate of .015% nine weeks after the lockdown. Still, let's stay locked down forever!

As Texas began reopening on May 1, reporters were flocking to Dallas and Houston and reporting live on city streets, donning face masks in open-air outdoors with no one near them, and no state order to do so. You'd think that SARS-CoV-2 was flying in the wind like snowflakes in a Michigan blizzard in January.

Restaurants were reopening with limited capacity, some retail stores for "takeout." CNN was making an argument that Texas should not reopen until they had a 14-day decline in cases. By May 1, we knew from studies already discussed that the actual number of "cases" was vastly higher in America and worldwide than any figures would state. You can see on the CNN screen the prominence that cases and deaths were given. No one discussed context.

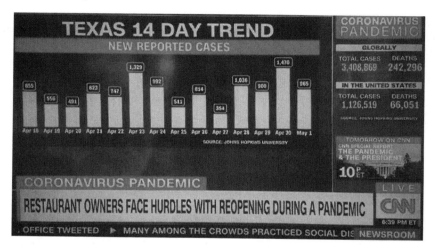

At this date, Texas had less than a thousand total COVID-19 deaths in a state home to nearly 30 million people. Around 1,900 people were in hospitals with COVID-19. The fatalities were 3 in 10,000 residents, nearly all with preexisting conditions or the elderly. That is in no way discounting those at risk. Rather, it's that we knew who was at risk and protect them while letting the rest of the populace get back to work and school.

On May 16, ABC News ran this headline: "*Texas cases of COVID-19 increasing by thousands since reopening; Texas has seen a steady rise in novel coronavirus cases and fatalities since reopening just over two weeks ago.*"[278] What Texas did realize in their "steady rise" was 58 COVID-19 deaths on May 14. Texas loses an average of 800 people every day. COVID-19 hospitalizations were flat since the reopening. Cases up, no change in hospitalizations. Where was that headline? Did the media understand what was happening?

Since the lockdowns began in March, about 48,000 people died in Texas to all-causes, and 1,340 to COVID-19. That's 3% of all deaths and .004% of the population to COVID-19. Is there any chance any reasonable person would have locked down 29MM people with that kind of result?

Another piece that ran on CNN in early May (below) was the debate on meat processing plants opening as many in plants already discussed tested positive for the virus. The theme was that President Trump was forcing plants to open against their wishes. What wasn't discussed was that no plant was forced to open.

One-hundred-fifteen meat processing plants across the country employ approximately 130,000 workers. Every single state had COVID-19 cases in those plants. Around 4,913 people from those plants tested positive for the virus (the testing was not completed for all 130,000), most were asymptomatic, and 20 of those lost their lives.[279] That fatality rate is .4% of the positive tests and .015% of all workers.

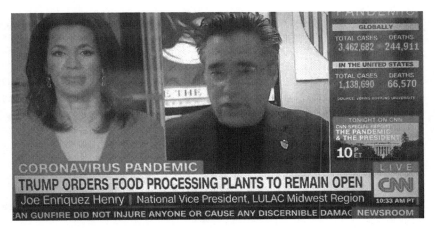

CNN and MSNBC were not the only cable networks showing inaccurate data reporting. Fox News and One America News opinion anchors were much more in favor of reopening than anchors and panelists on the other major cable and news networks. Would they have taken the opposite view if President Obama were in office? It seems unlikely that a populist at heart like Tucker Carlson would have resisted reopening states, schools and the economy given the data available. Even as Fox News opinion anchors were clamoring to get the country reopened, Fox News ran this on a May 2, 2020 broadcast:

Having grown up in the Detroit area, I was quickly drawn to the Wayne County data. At a glance it did not make sense, knowing the data and Detroit so well. Wayne County has 1.7 million residents including Detroiters, plus many other densely populated cities. Wayne County had 1,184 total COVID-19 deaths by that date. Doing some simple math, the actual number of COVID-19 deaths per 100,000 residents in Wayne County was 69. Fox News was reporting 968, incorrect by a factor of 14.

The data on-screen meant that 20,128 Wayne County residents died of COVID-19 in that one-month span, compared to the actual 1,184. If you were watching this data, particularly as a Detroiter, you'd never go outside nor support reopening. If instead, the reporting was 69 and that 90% of the fatalities were to people with preexisting conditions and the elderly and largely from nursing homes, you'd think we need to protect those vulnerable but the rest of the population should get back to normal. About 100,000 people in Michigan die every year.[280]

On May 4, a poll conducted by *The Washington Post* and the University of Maryland was released and below is a clip from a MSNBC broadcast. A high majority of people opposed opening just about everything. And why not? With the news circulated in just about every media outlet, it would take a grassroots awareness of gradual toe-dipping in the ocean to see the shark was not waiting in the waters.

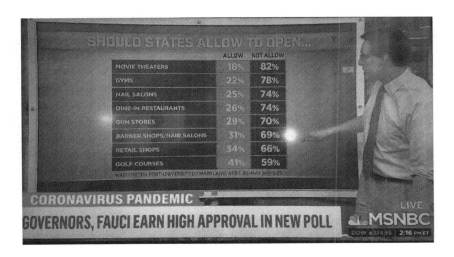

It's not surprising. Most media outlets became Jan Brady shouting, "Cases Cases Cases!" An ABC News/Ipsos poll on May 8 showed 92% of Democrats did not want the country reopened, to 35% Republicans.[281] Other results are below. We would still have a way to go for Americans to drive normalcy again, but it was inching its way forward compared to how most Americans felt a few weeks earlier.

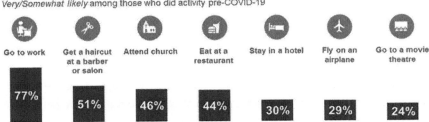

Majorities of Americans not ready to resume most activities, even if restrictions were lifted tomorrow

Most Americans would go to work, but they would forgo resuming most other public activities

If social distancing orders and restrictions on public activity were lifted tomorrow, how likely would you be to do each of the following?

% *Very/Somewhat likely* among those who did activity pre-COVID-19

Go to work	Get a haircut at a barber or salon	Attend church	Eat at a restaurant	Stay in a hotel	Fly on an airplane	Go to a movie theatre
77%	51%	46%	44%	30%	29%	24%

Q4. If social distancing orders and restrictions on public activity were lifted tomorrow, how likely would you be to do each of the following?

© 2020 Ipsos

With no restrictions, fewer than half were willing to go to the movies, travel, even go to church or out to dinner. However, practicality would set in. As life resumed and hospitalizations and deaths did not explode or even grow, would they gradually ease back to normal? Maybe. If the media did not dam up the facts? Definitely.

The Associated Press-NORC Center for Public Affairs Research conducted a poll on coronavirus issues including trust in the media.[282] The survey found (emphasis added):

- *"6 in 10 Americans say they regularly get information about COVID-19 from the news media. Half listen to state and local governments on a regular basis. About another 4 in 10 often look to the CDC. Fewer — about 3 in 10 — go to Trump regularly, with roughly as many listening to the president occasionally.*
- *Personal networks are less frequent sources for many Americans, though majorities get information about the virus from them at least some of the time. Twenty-eight percent regularly look to friends and family, with 43% occasionally going to them for information. Personal doctors and health care providers are used regularly by 18% of Americans and occasionally by 36%.*
- *While the news media is the most frequented source of information about the virus, it is one of the least trusted. **Only about a third say they have high trust in information about the virus from the news media.** Roughly another third have a moderate amount of trust.*
- *Three in 10 Americans say they use social media for coronavirus information regularly, with roughly the same share using it as a source on occasion. **Just about 1 in 10 say they have high levels of trust in coronavirus information from social media; nearly two-thirds report having little to none.**"*

While the poll indicates a low trust in the media, it was where everyone got their information. Even listening to state and local governments as half of the respondents did, that too is politicized. It's probably too much to get people to spend time visiting resources like *The Lancet* and *medRxiv* for unbiased data, though that would enlighten everyone on what was really happening with the pandemic. Still, if this pandemic has taught us anything, it's that any piece of news should be reconciled with two to three different varying sources to get clarity on any issue.

CHAPTER 19

SOCIAL COLLAPSE AMIDST THE CHAOS

By the end of April, about 2.6 billion people were through or were still under lockdowns for a matter of weeks. Below is a list of countries and the number of people per country.

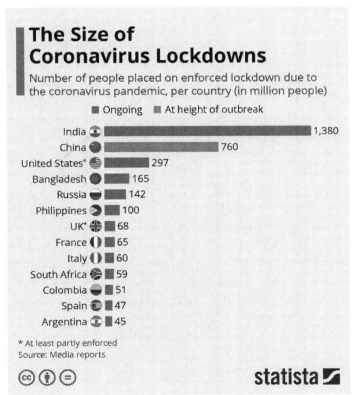

The Size of Coronavirus Lockdowns

Number of people placed on enforced lockdown due to the coronavirus pandemic, per country (in million people)

■ Ongoing ■ At height of outbreak

India	1,380
China	760
United States*	297
Bangladesh	165
Russia	142
Philippines	100
UK*	68
France	65
Italy	60
South Africa	59
Colombia	51
Spain	47
Argentina	45

* At least partly enforced
Source: Media reports

statista 🅉

The world had never seen a social lockdown like this. We know the impact the lockdowns had on the economy, but what about qualitative impacts? What effect did the lockdowns have on people's behavior, psychology, joy or depression?

Quarantining, social distancing and stay-at-home orders hit Americans much harder as a population than the coronavirus did. People are inherently social. People need to feel in control of their lives to feel freedom and peace.

Sit for a minute on your couch. You could probably do that comfortably for the duration of a movie. Now, as you're sitting on your couch, imagine a glass enclosure boxing you around your couch with a few feet of space to move around, the same as you might readjust while you're watching that movie. Would you still feel at peace watching the movie or would you become nervous knowing you did not have the freedom to move about? That anxiety was felt by millions of Americans during the COVID-19 lockdowns.

DOMESTIC CHALLENGES

Sixty-two million couples were in marriages in 2020 in the United States, representing 37% of all Americans. Many are very happily married and many are not. One survey stated 64% are "very happy" and in that same survey, just 19% are unhappy.[283] Dana Adam Shapiro wrote the book, *You Can Be Right or You Can Be Married*, and in it wrote that as few as 17% of couples are content with their partner.[284] In a lengthy survey in the UK, married couples rated their life satisfaction 9.9% higher than widows and widowers and nearly 9% happier than divorced or separated people. To be sure, being happily married is one of the most fulfilling experiences for most people.[285]

Regardless of the number, millions of Americans are in unhappy marriages and relationships. How would the lockdowns affect them, without diversions of going out, doing activities with same-gender friends, escaping to work and shopping?

A fascinating report published by *The Economist* about Chicago, Kansas City, Los Angeles, Memphis and New Orleans illustrates an inverse relationship during the lockdowns.[286] Traditional crimes (rape, break-ins, murder) went down and domestic violence went up. The United Nations Population Fund published an analysis on gender-based violence and interestingly, on the impact COVID-19 will have on unplanned pregnancies.[287]

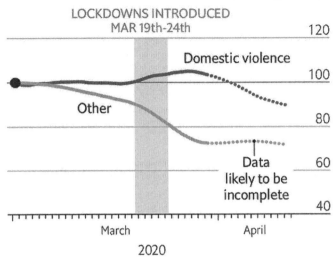

United States, reported crimes per day
Selected cities*, Mar 1st 2020=100, 7-day moving average

LOCKDOWNS INTRODUCED
MAR 19th-24th   120

Domestic violence   100

Other

80

Data
likely to be
incomplete   60

40

March   April

2020

Sources: Police and municipal records; Danish National
Domestic Violence Hotline (Lev Uden Vold)
The Economist

The prediction, global in nature, stated that stay-at-home orders will increase women's exposure to violent partners, coupled with economic stress and household tension. Another cause is delayed response help for victims in these situations. A 20% increase in domestic violence cases would result in 15 million more cases in just 2020.

Sadly, domestic violence seems to increase any time families spend more time together, like vacations and holidays. With more families contained than any time in American history, domestic violence would see a surge. Women and children are the predominant victims of domestic violence.

The Houston police received 300 more calls for domestic violence in March than they did in February, a 20% increase.[288] Even with more days in March, it's a huge increase at a time when the weather would be warming and in other times people would be spending more time outside, away from home, and kids' spring activities would be ramping up.

Charlotte, NC had 517 more calls in March 2020 than in March 2019, an 18% increase. Phoenix, AZ jumped a little in single digits. Nashville and surrounding areas in Tennessee received a 55% increase in hotline calls since the lockdowns. The United Nations refer to this as a "shadow pandemic." A similar hotline in England received 49% more calls for domestic/partner violence in just the period of the UK's lockdown.[289]

The Michigan Coalition to End Domestic and Sexual Violence said calls have increased to 393 in March and the first half of April in 2020, up from 189 the same time last year. Michigan's Domestic and Sexual Violence Prevention and Treatment Board has also seen a jump in help requests, although data are not yet available. In my hometown area of Oakland County, a Detroit suburb, domestic violence charges jumped 47% in the first two weeks of April year-over-year.[290]

In the UK, the abuse charity Refuge reported a "700% increase in calls to its helpline in a single day in April, while a separate helpline for perpetrators of domestic abuse seeking help to change their behavior received 25% more calls after the start of the COVID-19 lockdown."[291] In this report they cited that three times the number of women were killed by men during the lockdowns in April, though the absolute number was 14.

CHILDREN

Partners weren't the only ones suffering from increased domestic abuse. Child abuse was spiking up dramatically as well. The Rape, Abuse and Incest National Network (RAINN) has a hotline available for victims of child abuse. Partner abuse is one thing, an ugly thing, but child abuse has to be the most heinous crime committed. As a parent and baseball coach for a decade, it's hard to fathom being abusive to a child. RAINN received a 22% increase in calls from kids under 18 for sexual abuse, committed by someone within the family or someone living with the family.[292]

Kids were never demonstrated victims or transmitters of COVID-19. By removing kids from their activities, school, sports, they were removed from watchful eyes. They also prevented impatient parents from getting their "space," thus making them less patient in their time together.

Abusers might temper their abuse knowing the kids would be seen in school or elsewhere by others and therefore be exposed. With stress abound in families and knowing kids would be insulated, it makes logical sense the lockdown period would be more challenging for kids than many adults.

In a 2017 study by Dan Brown and Elisabetta De Cao called *The Impact of Unemployment on Child Abuse and Neglect in the United States*, they identified a correlation between unemployment and partner and child abuse.[293] More prevalent in poor than wealthier families, a 1% increase in unemployment led to a 25 % increase in neglect and a 12% increase in abuse. What would a 10% increase in unemployment do? Even with subsidized unemployment benefits, the results couldn't be good.

Angelina Jolie wrote in *Time Magazine* echoing this concern.[294] Jolie has been an advocate of the MeToo movement, and rights of children long before the COVID-19 pandemic struck. Charlize Theron donated $1MM to help with the victims of abuse.

The other callout they made was that with social distancing limitations, less money and less places to get them, contraceptive use would decline. The analysis provided a range of 325,000 to a million unplanned pregnancies in a low health service disruption, which it appears this will be globally, a few weeks in each country. Total abortions the second half of 2020 will likely see a sharp year-over-year increase.

CRIME

Finally, a good unintended good consequence of the COVID-19 pandemic! Violent crime went down, in some cities anyway. With people staying in and not going out, the pool of potential victims dropped dramatically. St. Louis had a 77% drop in murders in 2020 over 2019 by May. Atlanta saw a similar dip in violent crimes in April compared to the previous year. South Africa saw a near identical drop in murders as St. Louis had. South Africa also saw a drop in rapes from 700 to 101 year-over-year. Serious assault cases plummeted from 2,673 to 456, and murders fell from 326 to 94.[295]

Sioux City, Iowa saw a similar drop from January/February assaults to what was reported in April. With bars closed, bar brawls dropped to nothing. San Bernardino, California traditionally has a healthy crime rate. Property crimes dropped, rapes dropped, burglaries saw the biggest drop year-over-year, by a third. Vehicle thefts dropped.[296] Breaking the trend, Philadelphia saw a spike in murders in April 2020.

Chicago has been maybe the most violent city in America in the 2010's. Police there saw a 42% drop in drug arrests during the lockdowns.[297] With "customers" locked down, drug sellers along with all retailers lost their customer base. Fortunately, drug dealer subsidization was not part of the CARES Act. In a different twist, as part of Japan's $1T stimulus package, sex worker financial aid was provided. Down south, El Salvador saw a drop from a high of 600 killings per day to two a day during the pandemic. Crime dropped 84% in Peru.

Cincinnati had a very different experience. During the April lockdown, murder rose 115% compared to April the previous year, shootings were up 52% and robberies went up 31%. Not every city had this result, but that's an enormous increase in crime.[298]

The AP shared this insight into a Maryland entrepreneur. A Maryland man accused of operating a Darknet store selling prescription opioids boasted on his vendor page: "*Even with Corona Virus the shop is running at full speed.*" He told an undercover FBI agent he was just waiting for a shipment because "this corona virus shit is fucking up inventory," according to court documents.[299] One more supply chain challenge that the country had to overcome.

While India's lockdown was a travesty of epic proportions, a platinum lining was the drop in crime. Registered crimes in Delhi dropped from 3,416 to 1,890 year-over-year.[300] Molestations dropped, kidnappings dropped and robberies dropped, all nearly in half. With supply chains fractured and income sources dropping, it's almost surprising, unless the reporting of crimes dropped but actual ones still occurred. Car accidents dropped to zero in one Indian city, not seen before. And 98% of would-be cars on the road were no longer.

New York bucked this trend. New York City saw an increase in murders during the lockdown. Murders had doubled in April year-over-year and shootings were up 21% for the year. Murders in each week in April averaged about 10 compared to half that in the prior year. Five of 29 murders in New York were related to domestic violence for the first six weeks of the lockdown.[301] By May, shootings jumped sharply, quadrupling the second week of the month compared to the week prior.[302] Chicago later saw a huge rise in murders as May closed and into June.

SUICIDES

On March 25, 2020, President Trump made the comment that lockdowns and imminent high unemployment would cause more suicide deaths than the coronavirus. Like many things President Trump says, it was a bit of a hyperbolic statement. He was crucified for the statement by his critics. Still, there was merit to what he said.

Anyone who does not believe suicides will spike as a result of the lockdowns has to be living under a rock. Or, like most in the media, be enjoying a high six or seven-figure income during the lockdown.

When the financial crisis hit in 2007 and a recession ensued, suicides spiked by 10,000 over prior periods in America and Europe. Suicides are the tenth largest cause of death in America, claiming up to 50,000 lives a year. Mental health is an obvious reason why some choose to end their lives, but it's not the biggest reason. It's severe depression.

Large contributors to people committing suicide include job insecurity, losing a job, having a serious or chronic medical condition, being a victim of abuse and a lack of help resources for those seeking it. All those depressive conditions would be magnified during the pandemic and lockdown. The highest age bracket for suicides is 45-54 followed by the elderly over 80. More than three quarters of suicide victims are white compared to about half the population. Most commit suicide with a gun.[303]

WILX in Lansing, MI, reported an opinion based on conversations with front line healthcare workers in the Detroit-area that they expect those under stress and depression would provide a 32% increase in suicides over the pandemic and lockdown. Dr. Lorna Breen was the highest profile suicide during the pandemic. Breen was an ER doctor at New York-Presbyterian Allen Hospital in northern Manhattan. She was 49. She contracted the virus and recovered. If you've spent any time talking to physicians, they will tell you that working in the emergency room is the highest stress specialty in the field.[304]

The longer one is quarantined, the more likely one is to suffer from mental health, post-traumatic stress, anger and introversion. The over-under for COVID-19 symptoms to take hold is about 10 days according to one study. When SARS broke in 2003, we saw an increase in elderly suicides. With the elderly the second highest segment of suicides, and now facing greater isolation because they are the most vulnerable, they're balancing a fear of death because they are the most vulnerable and depression because they're isolated from families in many cases.[305] This will be important to watch in the latter months of 2020 and 2021.

Still think President Trump was off base in his remarks? Suicide hotlines experienced an 800% increase in calls since the lockdowns began. Former Congressman Patrick Kennedy, a Democrat, said, "The tragedy of COVID is it exacerbates this already prevalent mental health and addiction crisis. No one doubts that mental health and addiction is real. Every single American has been faced with a mental health issue in this COVID crisis, themselves, not just a family member, but themselves."[306]

In Australia, it may become true to life. Several medical experts reported that the lockdowns and economic carnage could result in an extra 1,500 suicide deaths a year over the next five years, where Australia typically sees 3,000 suicides a year. *The Daily Mail's* headline says it all, "The Silent Covid-19 Death Toll: Far more Australians will kill themselves because of the Coronavirus Lockdown than those who die of the virus."[307] Sydney University's Brain and Mind Centre predicted four times more would die from suicide than from COVID-19.

Results from a national survey found 35% of those surveyed felt anxious or depressed, with 42% of those attributing it to job reduction or loss. Fifty-three percent of people responding to the survey said they were in moderate distress, with 27% in high distress. One out of four people reported binge drinking at least once a week. One out of five people said they took prescription drugs for non-medical reasons.[308]

Association between income inequality and suicide rate in the United States

Suicide rate for working age adults vs income inequality

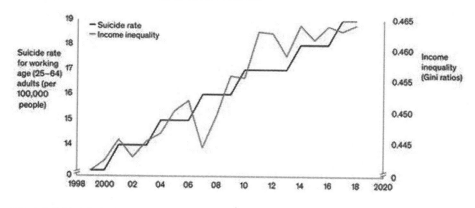

Source: CDC WISQARS, 2020; U.S. Census Bureau, Current Population Survey, 1968 to 2019 Annual Social and Economic Supplements (CPS ASEC)

McKinsey
& Company

A CDC analysis above draws direct lines between income inequality and suicides. With what may grow to 40 million people out of work, many non-Covid-19 illnesses untreated for weeks, it seems impossible not to see a suicide rise in America from 2020 to 2022.

DEATHS OF DESPAIR

The Robert Graham Center for Policy Studies in Family Medicine and Primary Care conducted analysis on the impact of the lockdowns, depression, job loss and fear on suicide levels.[309] Their findings are below. "Three factors, already at work, are exacerbating deaths of despair: unprecedented economic failure paired with massive unemployment, mandated social isolation for months and possible residual isolation for years."

In 2018, there were 181,686 "deaths of despair," from alcohol, drugs or suicide. They estimated that based on unemployment up and isolation growing, the lockdowns could result in 65,598 more deaths of despair annually for several years. Contextualize that with the pandemic – collateral deaths from this and untreated non-COVID-19 health conditions could far eclipse COVID-19 deaths.

They based their data on actual results that occurred in the wake of the Great Recession 12 years before COVID-19 reached America. With unemployment up 10 points in a month from the lockdowns, they predicted deaths that might eclipse actual COVID-19 fatalities. Combine this with expected fatalities from untreated non-COVID-19 patients and it's very possible that collateral deaths could exceed real COVID-19 deaths.

The chart below represents possibilities based on 1-1.6% increases in unemployment. What about a 10% increase? The incremental projections below are very small compared to the very high unemployment from the lockdowns. Projecting that may be off the charts.

Table. Possible Additional Deaths of COVID-19 Recession on Deaths of Despair, Alternative Scenarios								
Percent Change in Mortality with One Point Increase in Unemployment								
	1% increase			1.3% increase			1.6% increase		
	Slow	Medium	Fast	Slow	Medium	Fast	Slow	Medium	Fast
2020	9,859	9,333	8,343	12,817	12,133	10,846	15,774	14,932	13,349
2021	18,347	16,103	12,209	23,851	20,934	15,871	29,355	25,765	19,534
2022	15,879	11,840	5,832	20,642	15,392	7,581	25,406	18,944	9,331
2023	13,410	8,025	1,261	17,434	10,433	1,639	21,457	12,841	2,017
2024	10,394	3,973	-	13,512	5,164	-	16,630	6,356	-
2025	7,651	870	-	9,947	1,131	-	12,242	1,392	-
2026	7,103	316	-	9,234	411	-	11,365	506	-
2027	5,732	-	-	7,451	-	-	9,171	-	-
2028	4,086	-	-	5,312	-	-	6,538	-	-
2029	3,812	-	-	4,956	-	-	6,099	-	-
Total	96,273	50,460	27,644	125,155	65,598	35,937	154,037	80,735	44,230

Types of Recovery: Slow—Same as Great Recession; Medium—Twice as Fast; Fast—Four Times as fast.

Above chart: Well Being Trust & The Robert Graham Center Analysis: The COVID Pandemic Could Lead to 75,000 Additional Deaths from Alcohol and Drug Misuse and Suicide: https://wellbeingtrust.org/areas-of-focus/policy-and-advocacy/reports/projected-deaths-of-despair-during-covid-19/

DISTANCE LEARNING

On April 29, 2020, while writing this book, I was texting with one of my friends about school in the wake of the lockdowns and how kids were sent home to learn remotely. Her son is a bright young man at the Air Force Academy studying engineering. I asked her how it was going for him, and she texted me a real-time video of her son asleep in bed next to his laptop, which was running an online class at the same time. It's a funny story and the video is hilarious, but how were kids coping with distance learning?

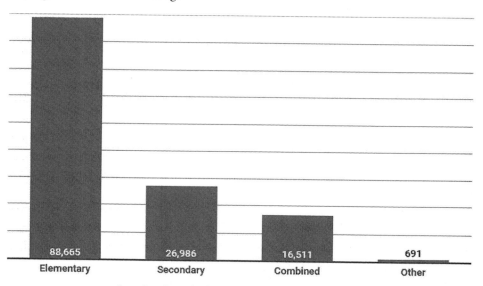

Source: https://www.edweek.org/ew/issues/education-statistics/index.html

This is how many pre-college schools there are in America. Take a quick look at how many kids are enrolled in school in the top 10 ISDs in the country (below).[310] Nearly 55 million kids are enrolled in school, from pre-kindergarten through high school. Close to 20 million more are enrolled in college or university classes.

RANK	DISTRICT NAME	STATE	ENROLLMENT
1	New York City	NY	984,462
2	Los Angeles	CA	633,621
3	Chicago	IL	378,199
4	Miami-Dade	FL	357,249

5	Clark County	NV	326,953
6	Broward County	FL	271,852
7	Houston	TX	216,106
8	Hillsborough County	FL	214,386
9	Orange County	FL	200,674
10	Palm Beach County	FL	192,721

Seventy-five million kids and young adults went from structured, mostly instructor-led teaching to online classes, Zoom deliveries, and in some cases, distance learning. Worldwide, 1.5 billion students were out of school, all to a virus that had no measurable effect on kids. It would test parents and students alike. For kids from pre-K to late middle school, parents would have to take the lead on helping with lessons, while enduring the stress of their lost job, or working from home, and isolation. It had all the makings of a new Calgon commercial.

Tutoring was hugely compromised for those who could afford it, since lockdowns prevented that. With my son home from college, he placed an advertisement to tutor, something he did his last couple of years in high school. He got only one response, an inquiry for a FaceTime session in algebra. We were stunned, thinking he'd be inundated with requests, until we realized the lockdowns and fear of the virus prevented people from seeking tutorial help.

Families were cooped up like never before. Work-from-home responsibilities competed for quiet space and reliable Internet connectivity for many. Most parents are not well-equipped to bridge the teaching gap. Kids with any kind of learning disability or lack of motivation were going to suffer.

The Los Angeles Unified School District is the second-largest school system. Into late April, a fourth of all students had not logged into online classes at all. That was for high school students. It was worse for elementary students. In Baltimore, only a quarter of students had their own laptops. Imagine the crunch of a poor family sharing a laptop or not having one, being out of work and faced with an extra $500 expenditure.[311]

Atlanta has an estimated 6,000 students without computers. Marginalized communities suffered the most. It's the saddest thing about this situation, where the weakest suffered the most both medically and in education. It really was Darwinism in action. More than half of Louisiana's school districts said that half their students don't even have internet connectivity at home let alone a computer.

For all the time cable news debated President Trump's comment about disinfectants at the height of all this, you'd never see a story on education challenges covered. Had there been media pressure to reopen schools, no doubt schools would have resumed in May in many states.

Most schools opted not to try to teach new material. Most fall semesters in high school begin with a few weeks of previous year review in classes where the material of one year builds on the previous. Schools were floating ideas of longer school days or beginning earlier in August. The latter is a viable option, but the former would never work. There is just a limit any person has per day or session to absorb information before there's a diminishing return.

There are no great options. Parents and kids alike may not embrace any day or school year extensions given family obligations and activities. This breakdown will never make big headlines but after the overall economic disruption and delayed non-COVID-19 medical treatments, it's the biggest casualty of the lockdowns. Given that hospitals were empty and every day that passed by late April had cases going up and hospitalizations going down, it's somewhere between reckless and insane that schools did not reopen. Few if any cases were uncovered in the world by May 1 where a child passed the virus on to an adult or had any otherwise-healthy child died from COVID-19.

Colleges gave students the option for an earned grade or simply a pass/fail grade, and they got to decide that after their earned grades were released. That seemed like a reasonable compromise. Also, preventive litigation. If learning delivery were compromised, a good argument could be made about the schools' participation if students' grades suffered.

I talked to a roundtable of college students about this. The bright ones disagreed and said it's just a matter of how much you wanted it, self-motivation. However, it's easy to say that when you're a gifted student. Most students benefit greatly from the structure school provides. Dozens of schools were sued by the summer of 2020 for not giving a tuition break due to delivery moving from live instructor led to online.

The Network for Public Education conducted a survey in April 2020 with parents, teachers and school administrators responding. The survey asked about both how online delivery was working quantitatively and how teachers and parents felt qualitatively.[312]

TEACHER RESPONSES

- More than 60% of the teachers responded that they were spending six hours or less per day on teaching, planning and grading.

- More than 70% of the work done was not being graded, meaning it was pass/fail, undetermined or nothing.
- Online work comprised more than 80% of the lessons, connect that dot to the number of kids without access or computers.
- Around 64% of the teachers were doing video conferences once or week or more with students. Still, it would take a self-motivated child or parent to bother.
- The teachers said two-thirds of their students were struggling with adjusting to online work.
- When asked how they felt about distance learning as a teacher (responses not mutually exclusive):
  - 57% overwhelmed
  - 44% anxious
  - 32% struggling
  - 29% supported
  - 25% lonely
  - 14% not supported
- More than half felt their students would be behind whenever school would resume.
- Around 60% of the students were not engaging each day in lesson plans.

PARENT RESPONSES

- Parents from all different makeups responded with the majority suburban, nearly all working from home, with the majority having high school age kids:
- More than 80% said their kids were spending 1-4 hours a day on schoolwork.
- About 90% said they had a laptop and Internet connectivity.
- About 90% said their kids were conferencing with their teachers.
- Only 20% said their kids were struggling to adjust to distance learning.
- When asked what their children miss most about school closures, they responded:
  - 83% miss their friends
  - 60% missed their teachers
  - 59% missed sports and extracurricular activities
  - 39% were lonely

One comment on this is that the connection between parents who responded to this survey would be more inclined to have more online resources and be hands-on parents. It was an online survey, not a random sampling. The teacher comments are telling. Schools couldn't reopen fast enough. Alas, classrooms remained empty for the 2019-2020 school year in almost all states.

Meanwhile, many kids 15 and older were allowed to work at grocery and other retail stores that were open. So, they could work but not go to school? Think about that. In May, in New Brunswick, Canada, middle and high school students were recruited for lobster processing to fill the gap of foreign workers unavailable. Why not? School was out, sort of.

On May 6, 2020, Australian states began the process of getting their kids back to school. They cited a few studies, all which pointed to low infection and transmission with younger people. Britain's NSW conducted a study in April of 735 students and 128 school staff in close contact with 18 known positive cases. No one within the school staff caught it from those 18 cases. A study out of the Netherlands reported children are less likely to get infected by the virus from adults.[313] Not a single study has reported anything but that kids are not measurably affected by the virus, in this segment of the population SARS-COV-2 is much less dangerous than influenza.

On May 5, *The New York Times* published a piece warning that "cases could soar" if schools were reopened.[314] It was an opinion piece that refuted all known data at this time. The supposition is that keeping schools closed reduces a "surge by 40 to 60%." It was one more panic and fear-inducing media piece that was not borne in data. Overwhelming data from all over the world demonstrated that children were both not measurably vulnerable to infection nor transmission. Children simply weren't getting sick. Unlike flu viruses, which spread most often through children, they were somewhere between unable to transmit the virus because their load was so low or weren't transmitting it if they were capable.

Sometimes you need to step back at a macro level of data analysis. At the time the piece above was published, deaths had reached a 35-day low, and hospitalizations had fallen off. The macro logic said it was time to get kids back to school, the big-picture data was irrefutable.

By early May, schools were opening in France, Switzerland, Australia, China, Denmark, Germany, Israel. Japan and Norway had reopened schools already. Sweden never shut their lower grades down.

On May 7, schools began reopening in Idaho and Montana. All other states had cancelled school for the school year, but these states moving first was a huge first step to normalization. Great work to Governors Brad Little and Steve Bullock!

On June 17, 2020, the Hospital for Sick Children, Canada's pediatric medical center set back to school guidelines for the fall. They called out children are at low risk for infection and transmission and recommended kids go back to school without face masks.[315]

SPECIAL NEEDS

The challenge was exasperated for children with special needs. The Philadelphia school system identifies 17% of their students as special needs, Illinois about 14%. Students with autism were relegated largely to parents shouldering that load, while balancing their own work, and patience. Special-needs kids are most successful with routines and those had disappeared. How practical is it for a special needs child of any level to sit in front of a computer and learn?

Parents are barely equipped to help average to gifted students with their work from eighth or ninth grade on, myself included. A neighbor of mine is a physician and he was unable to help his tenth grader with math, though he excelled at it in his day. Most parents would be stretched with the education burden, even in the discipline and motivation. That would rise another level with parents of kids with special needs. It usually takes a team to usher along learning for special-needs kids, plus with specialized resources and learning tools.

With COVID-19 hospitalizations down to a small fraction of capacity, services like these would be closed. It's no one's fault, a casualty of the pandemic. But wait just a moment. It may be someone's fault. These state and local re-openings would linger much longer than it took to shut everything down.

Meanwhile, hospitals were practically empty of COVID-19 patients.

CHAPTER 20

AGAINST THE WALL

Madonna stood on the main stage near the Washington Mall the day after the 2017 inauguration and said, "*Yes, I am outraged. Yes, I have thought an awful lot about blowing up the White House... but I choose love.*" Ashley Judd complemented that, telling the huge crowd, "*I am a nasty woman. I'm not as nasty as a man who looks like he bathes in Cheeto dust. A man whose words are a distraction to America; Electoral College-sanctioned hate speech contaminating this national anthem.*"[316]

Scarlet Johansson was bit more measured, saying, "*President Trump, I did not vote for you. That said... I want to be able to support you, but first I ask that you support me.*" These celebrities speaking at the Women's March in 2017 were not happy about the 2016 election results, nor were the close to half a million mostly women there or the few million protesting around the country.

In 1913, 5,000 women marched in front of the White House while a half million watched them protest for the right to vote. It's hard to believe that just a hundred years ago, women weren't allowed to vote. In the summer of 1963, 250,000 people gathered, mostly black Americans but about a quarter white, to protest the inequalities black people were facing in America. A man named Martin Luther King Jr. told the crowd, "*I have a dream [that] my four little children will one day live in a nation where they will not be judged by the color of their skin but by the content of their character.*" It became the most famous protest quote in American history.

Protesting is one of the healthiest facets of American politics and culture. We achieve greatness when we stretch and pull each other to policies that affect most people in the most beneficial way. A government with strictly conservative policies or strictly liberal ones would never work for long in America.

If you don't agree with a March for Life protest, you may appreciate the benefit of at least discouraging very late term of partial birth abortions. If you don't agree with the Women's March, you may reflect back to the women's march of 1913 and how archaic women not voting looks today. You may not agree with everything Madonna said on stage that day, but you should fully appreciate her right to speak, and even her flair for delivery.

As the lockdowns continued for weeks, from March 2020 into the summer, many people started getting agitated. Americans were patient for a while, no one knew what would happen and they'd seen a lot of activity in Italy, France and New York. After three weeks or so, when no COVID-19 wave of hospitalizations hit most states, some started second guessing the lockdowns. As dissention grew, some state governors doubled down on their lockdown orders and even tightened them. Something was going to have to give.

WHO PROTESTS

More often than not, liberal mindsets tend to protest more than conservative ones. That's not a commentary. According to a Gallup poll in 2018, several findings were illuminated:

- 36% of Americans report having felt the urge to protest
- 60% of liberals and 21% of conservatives have felt the urge to protest
- Women's rights are the most cited reason to protest

Of those with the urge to protest the survey found[317]:

PARTY

Republican	21%
Independent	37%
Democrat	51%

POLITICAL IDEOLOGY

Conservative	21%
Moderate	36%
Liberal	60%

Protesters against the lockdowns this time would lean almost exclusively to conservatives, whether in Democrat or Republican-led states.

MICHIGAN

On April 10, Governor Gretchen Whitmer expanded Michigan's stay-at-home order, prohibiting Michiganders from visiting family or friends with exceptions for providing care, and preventing residents from traveling between different residences they may own. Michigan's dense population resides in the southeast, but many have homes in rural areas, around the Great Lakes, and getaway spots like Charlevoix and Traverse City in the north.

The order included a ban on use of motorboats, golf, and sales of carpeting, flooring, furniture, garden supplies or paint. It banned people from moving between homes in the state. Garden supplies banned from purchase at Home Depot or Ace Hardware? Paint? When you're locked down for weeks and prohibited from some DIY projects? Many would drive to Ohio for those things.

Residents congregated at an in-vehicle protest on April 15, driving to the capital in Lansing, MI. Thousands of people in cars and on foot protested the strict orders, the firsts of many protests against what some would see as an infringement on their constitutional rights.

Michigan House speaker, Lee Chatfield, posted on Twitter on April 11, *"Non-essential in Michigan: Lawn care, construction, fishing if boating with a motor, realtors, buying seeds, home improvement equipment and gardening supplies. Essential in Michigan: Marijuana, lottery and alcohol. Let's be safe and reasonable. Right now, we're not."*

Federal House Representative Justin Amash of Michigan was a former Republican and President Trump's greatest Republican critic in Congress. He tweeted this on Twitter following Whitmer's order, *"As a federal official, I do my best to stay out of state politics, but I have a constitutional duty to ensure states don't trample on the rights of the people. @GovWhitmer's latest order goes too far and will erode confidence in her leadership. She should immediately reassess it."*

Whitmer responded, saying, *"In World War II, there weren't people lining up at the Capitol to protest the fact that they had to drop everything they were doing and build planes or tanks or ration food."*[318] But this was not World War II. Hospitals all over Michigan were empty outside Wayne, Oakland and Macomb counties and all of them were hemorrhaging money. Health care workers in Michigan and even in the Detroit-area were being laid off or working reduced hours.

On April 30, Governor Whitmer extended the lockdown to May 28, with many states already loosening up. Whitmer explained, *"COVID-19 is an enemy that has taken the lives of more Michiganders than we lost during the Vietnam War.*

While some members of the legislature might believe this crisis is over, common sense and all of the scientific data tells us we're not out of the woods yet."[319]

However, scientific data was telling us that 99% of the people infected recovered, and less a few outliers, a very identifiable group of people were vulnerable to COVID-19. Michigan did have the third highest number of fatalities of any state, almost 4,000 at this time, behind New York and New Jersey. The graphic below shows Michigan's concentration of fatalities in the Detroit-area. The darkest county is Wayne, and the other two darker counties are Macomb and Oakland. The balance of the state was much less affected.

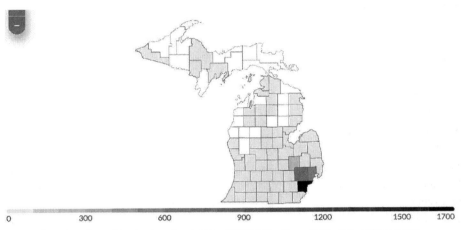

Source: https://www.clickondetroit.com/news/michigan/2020/03/25/tracking-covid-19-cases-by-michigan-county/

The next graphic illustrates the age distribution of cases and deaths in Michigan. Interestingly, a much higher percentage of cases were in younger people and the fatalities were weighted heavily with those older, something we saw all over the world. Of the cases at this time, about 40% were in those over 60 while 85% of the fatalities were in the same grouping. What agitated Michiganders is that knowing this, why not isolate and protect that segment of people and let the rest rebuild their lives? A million and a half people in Michigan were out of work.

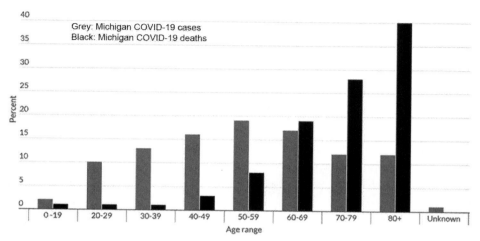

Source: https://www.clickondetroit.com/news/local/2020/03/31/tracking-michigan-covid-19-cases-by-age-range/

On the day Whitmer extended the lockdown another month, the most demonstrative spectacle of citizen protesting against any state lockdown occurred in Lansing, MI. Hundreds showed up at the state capital to protest the extended order, and the protest took a turn not seen yet. Some protesters were carrying rifles. No violence occurred, it's not clear if any of the weapons were loaded or just to make a statement.

A few hundred protesters were allowed in the capital building, calling for their constitutional rights and some were referencing the governor as Hitler. Check out some pictures online, it was quite a scene.

Whitmer said the protests depicted the worst in racism, with at least some brandishing confederate flags, nooses and allegedly Nazi symbols in addition to rifles. She was right in calling out the extreme messaging of some of the protesters. It's amazing to see any symbols of nooses and Nazis today. For any protesters that do not know it, it's very counterproductive to the message. When those symbols are seen, no other message matters. Thank you, Madonna, for not bringing the Nazis into your protest.

On May 6, Republican state legislators filed suit against Governor Whitmer alleging her extension of emergency declarations the previous week by executive order illegal, "absurd," unconstitutional and "nonsensical." Opposition in the state was asking the Michigan Court of Claims for an immediate ruling declaring that Whitmer's emergency orders, including her stay-at-home and business closure mandates, are "invalid and unenforceable" because the Legislature did not extend her emergency authority.[320]

On May 14, Michigan protesters, some with guns again, took a third run at the state capital. On a wet, rainy Thursday, a few hundred protesters gathered for the third time to end the stay at home order. One protest sign read, "Whitmer is the Virus" while another showed a poster of the governor with a Hitler-mustache drawn in. The lockdowns continued.

CALIFORNIA

After five weeks of shutdown, San Clemente, in Orange County, voted to open their beaches. April 25 was unseasonably warm in southern California. Tens of thousands of people showed up on beaches in Orange County making headlines nationally. People were getting antsy and ready to move on. They'd been cooped up for more than a month. Nothing was happening in California, there was no hospitalization wave, and some demonstrated they were ready to get back to normal.

On April 24, Los Angeles Mayor Eric Garcetti said, "*There is a direct correlation between what you do this weekend and how long this will take and how many lives we will lose. If you stay home this weekend, our case numbers will drop, and we will stop the spread of this virus.*"[321] The following weekend, Governor Newsom closed all Orange County beaches. Hospitals were still empty, and each day new evidence of more positive tests and fewer casualties was realized.

In response to the beachgoers the weekend of April 25, Governor Newsom would issue a closure of just Orange County beaches the next weekend, for May 2-3. Only Orange County beaches would be closed for the weekend. That weekend a few thousand protesters gathered at Huntington Beach to express their displeasure at the governor's order. In addition, local governments at Huntington Beach and Dana Point began a legal challenge against both the governor and the state, as well as a restraining order.

Still, on this date hospitals were empty and California's fatality rate was 58 COVID-19 deaths per one million people. Millions of people were out of work in California, young people at no real risk and yet the governor was now doubling down on principle, as science had left his side.

On Monday, April 28, more protesters gathered in Orange County with some holding "Vote Newsom Out" signs. The governor responded to the beach protests saying restrictions would increase after the citizen defiance. A friend in California (he's liberal, not conservative) said it felt like he was a kid again and had been grounded for weeks, decided to get out to see some friends on a street corner and as punishment his parents reset his grounding.

On May 4, with either reality or pressure setting in, Governor Newsom followed Texas and sloooowly loosened retail restrictions, manufacturing restrictions, and loosened even more in rural counties and allow many counties to set their own guidelines. What took a day to shut down would take months to get back to normal in California, all while hospitals were basically free of COVID-19 emergencies.

On May 8, local leaders of Yuba, Sutter and Modoc counties lifted restrictions and allowed gyms, restaurants, shopping malls, hair salons and other businesses to open their doors again, ahead of the state's plans. While I began looking for property in those counties, Governor Newsom threatened those counties with withholding disaster assistance funding unless they complied with the state's orders. At this point, it became a power play. The California general ordered his troops to walk single file off El Cap and thank goodness some in the company refused.

It became an odyssey rather than protective measures against a pandemic that was threatening all Californians. California was barely affected in hospitalizations and fatalities, and half of those came from nursing homes, in part because the state ordered those facilities to take COVID-19 patients. If every resident of California knew all the data, Sacramento would have been overrun with protests.

Voters perked up on May 12, flipping a special election Democrat House seat to a Republican. The November election may end less a referendum on President Trump than who was for and against the lockdowns.

The same situation was repeated in Pennsylvania on May 11. Local leaders opened their cities and counties and the governor threatened them with withholding relief funds if they dissented. Power plays abound and the lockdowns fractured. The data wasn't supporting continued lockdowns. The troops were revolting.

ILLINOIS

Illinois was not an early state to begin reopening. On April 23 Governor J.B. Pritzker extended the state's stay at home order through May 30. Illinois State Representative Darren Bailey sued the governor and in what must have been a scene out of the TV show, *Suits*, was granted a restraining order. The order was for only himself unfortunately, the people of Illinois would have to wait.

On May 1, as Texas was reopening and people were shopping at malls in Atlanta, agitated Illinoisans began their second protest in a week. Hundreds gathered at the

Thompson Center in Chicago and the state capital to rally. Counter protesters demonstrated to remain locked down as well. Unlike Michigan, no reports of armed protesters appeared. A Nazi slogan, "Arbeit Macht Frei" (work sets you free), was seen on a protest sign. The woman holding the sign said she was Jewish and not a Nazi but was rather protesting Nazi-like government oppression. May protesters please get the message that nothing good comes from Nazi references at demonstrations? Ever.

On May 5, Governor Pritzker released "Restore Illinois," a detailed plan specifying the criteria for a phase 1-5 restoration.[322] To reach phase three, when nonessential businesses could resume, but still no gyms open, dining in, social distancing required with face masks, the following metrics would ALL have to be achieved:

- "At or under a 20% positivity rate and increasing no more than 10 percentage points over a 14-day period
- No overall increase (i.e. stability or decrease) in hospital admissions for COVID-19-like illness for 28 days
- Available surge capacity of at least 14% of ICU beds, medical and surgical beds, and ventilators
- Testing available in region regardless of symptoms or risk factors
- Tracing: Begin contact tracing and monitoring within 24 hours of diagnosis for more than 90% of cases in region"

If these rules did not bend, Illinoisans would be in for a long summer. Perhaps not all Illinois residents, however. During the stay-at-home order, the governor's wife flew to Florida to spend her time at their $12MM home in a state with lighter lockdowns.

In one other movie-like Illinois scene, Chicago Mayor Lori Lightfoot left the stay-at-home order to get her hair cut at the height of the rush in America in early April. Her stylist posted photos with the mayor on Facebook and thanked her for the *"pleasure of giving Mayor Lightfoot a hair trim."* The mayor defended the trim, saying, *"I'm the public face of this city. I'm on national media and I'm out in the public eye. I'm a person who, I take my personal hygiene very seriously, as I said I felt like I needed to have a haircut. I'm not able to do that myself."* Apparently, it's not just kids that need to be reminded that not everything belongs on social media.

NEW YORK

The New York City-area was hit in a way no other city or state was, and so their responses were definitely more understandable than those with low hospitalizations and fatalities. Still, by May, with other states moving on and New York seeing a steep decline in all things COVID-19, some residents were itchy to get back to normal.

On May 5, Mayor de Blasio banned any protests against the government policies. The city claimed that protests violated social distancing rules. On May 6, Governor Cuomo shared that two-thirds of all New York COVID-19 fatalities were transmitted in the home. The data doesn't support outdoor transmission of the virus, and most in New York who died caught it at home or in a nursing home. Still, the tight measures would go beyond the actual data.

TEXAS

Texas, the second largest state and economy in the country, led the way to reopening. Georgia announced first, but with Texas's size and stature, Governor Greg Abbott became a face of reopening. The last weekend in April, hundreds of protesters gathered at the capital in Austin at a "You Can't Close America Rally." Shouts of, "*Let us work!*" "*Put this on TV!*" and "*Fire Fauci!*" were heard. If Governor Abbott was listening, he had to be thinking "*I'm trying! Give me a few days, I promise we'll get this done.*" There was no question that during the shutdowns Governor Abbott and Lt. Governor Dan Patrick thought the lockdowns were too much.

In the highest-profile arrest and jailing in Texas in recent memory, Shelley Luther was guilty of opening her salon before the May 8 date allowed by Texas order. Luther closed her salon on March 22 like everyone else. On April 24, police officers visited her salon, issued her a citation and told her to close. Her salon was open but was respecting social distancing.

Luther did not and was arrested and arraigned on May 5. The Dallas judge gave her the option to apologize and admit wrongdoing and she would not be fined or serve time in jail. She declined on principle and said she would not apologize for opening her business to feed her children. She went immediately to a sheriff's jail to serve her one-week term. Lsuther explained to the judge, "*I have to disagree with you, sir, when you say that I'm selfish, because feeding my kids is not selfish. If you think the law's more important than kids getting fed, then please go ahead with your decision. But I am not going to shut the salon.*"

The story took a happy turn for Luther. She was out after two days served. Supporters set up a GoFundMe page and she was hailed a hero by many in the community. It's unlikely there will be an empty seat in her salon any time soon.

TESLA AND ELON MUSK

Many small businesses revolted from the shutdown orders and reopen. Shelley Luther was one of those, but there were many more. Karl Manke is a barber in Owosso, a very small town in Michigan. He decided to reopen his shop and a judge denied the state's request to issue a restraining order against him. All the businesses that revolted were small businesses during the lockdowns, no major corporations had made any waves. Until Elon Musk.

Tesla operates a plant in Fremont, California. Tesla also has a plant in China that was locked down and restarted, so Musk had been through this already. Musk was a vocal opponent of the lockdowns for much of April 2020 and reached his boiling point the second week of May, when California's lockdowns did not lighten up. California Governor Newsom issued an order allowing manufacturing to reopen on May 6 but Alameda County would not permit Tesla to reopen at the state-required 30% capacity.

Musk sued Alameda County over the continued shutdown and also threatened to move their headquarters from there to Texas.[323] Musk is a passionate genius, self-made and possesses an extremely high tolerance for risk. If anyone would be the first CEO to go through the wall, it would be Musk.

Time will reveal if other companies will threaten or actually leave the states that implemented stricter lockdown measure for those with lighter measures. Many believe Texas will see a boon over the next few years as companies become dissatisfied with their home states' policies during the lockdown. Even Bernie Sanders supporter Joe Rogan went off on California policies during a May show and pondered relocation to Texas.

RED AND BLUE REACTIONS

As protests to the lockdowns got momentum, *The New York Times* ran, "Conservatives Fuel Protests Against Coronavirus Lockdowns" as their report on the resistance.[324] Was it just conservatives protesting? Was there a clear difference between what was happening in predominately Democrat-voting states compared to Republican-voting states? And if so, why?

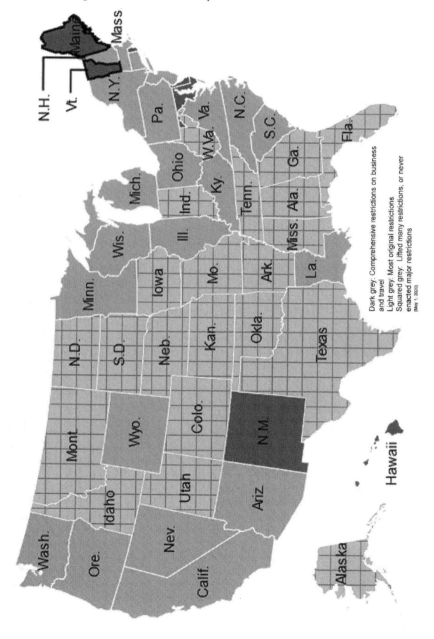

Dark grey: Comprehensive restrictions on business and travel
Light grey: Most original restrictions
Squared grey: Lifted many restrictions, or never enacted major restrictions
(May 1, 2020)

Below is each state governor, their party and their lockdown measures in May:

STATE	GOVERNOR	POLITICAL PARTY	LOCKDOWN MEASURE
California	Gavin Newsom	Democrat	Tight
Colorado	Jared Polis	Democrat	Loose
Connecticut	Ned Lamont	Democrat	Tight
Delaware	John C. Carney Jr.	Democrat	Tight
Hawaii	David Ige	Democrat	Tight
Illinois	J.B. Pritzker	Democrat	Tight
Kansas	Laura Kelly	Democrat	Loose
Kentucky	Andy Beshear	Democrat	Tight
Louisiana	John Bel Edwards	Democrat	Tight
Maine	Janet T. Mills	Democrat	Tight
Michigan	Gretchen Whitmer	Democrat	Tight
Minnesota	Tim Walz	Democrat	Tight
Montana	Steve Bullock	Democrat	Loose
Nevada	Steve Sisolak	Democrat	Tight
New Jersey	Phil Murphy	Democrat	Tight
New Mexico	Michelle Lujan Grisham	Democrat	Tight
New York	Andrew Cuomo	Democrat	Tight
North Carolina	Roy Cooper	Democrat	Tight
Oregon	Kate Brown	Democrat	Tight
Pennsylvania	Tom Wolf	Democrat	Tight
Rhode Island	Gina Raimondo	Democrat	Tight
Virginia	Ralph Northam	Democrat	Tight
Washington	Jay Inslee	Democrat	Tight
Wisconsin	Tony Evers	Democrat	Tight
Alabama	Kay Ivey	Republican	Loose
Alaska	Mike Dunleavy	Republican	Loose
Arizona	Doug Ducey	Republican	Tight
Arkansas	Asa Hutchinson	Republican	Loose

Florida	Ron DeSantis	Republican	Loose
Georgia	Brian Kemp	Republican	Loose
Idaho	Brad Little	Republican	Loose
Indiana	Eric Holcomb	Republican	Loose
Iowa	Kim Reynolds	Republican	Loose
Maryland	Larry Hogan	Republican	Tight
Massachusetts	Charles D. Baker	Republican	Tight
Mississippi	Tate Reeves	Republican	Loose
Missouri	Mike Parson	Republican	Loose
Nebraska	Pete Ricketts	Republican	Loose
New Hampshire	Chris Sununu	Republican	Tight
North Dakota	Doug Burgum	Republican	Loose
Ohio	Richard Michael DeWine	Republican	Tight
Oklahoma	Kevin Stitt	Republican	Loose
South Carolina	Henry McMaster	Republican	Tight
South Dakota	Kristi L. Noem	Republican	Loose
Tennessee	Bill Lee	Republican	Loose
Texas	Greg Abbott	Republican	Loose
Utah	Gary Herbert	Republican	Loose
Vermont	Phil Scott	Republican	Loose
West Virginia	Jim Justice	Republican	Tight
Wyoming	Mark Gordon	Republican	Loose

Of 24 Democrat governors, 21 maintained tight restrictions, or 88%. Of 26 Republican governors, 19 loosened restrictions, or 73%. The actions taken to maintain or loosen restrictions was highly correlated to party lines. Politics was driving the lockdowns at this point, while science and data were sitting in the back seat looking out the window. The November election may end up more a referendum on state policies during the pandemic versus a referendum on President Trump.

CHAPTER 21

AFTER ACTION REVIEW

The COVID-19 pandemic resulted in the greatest public policy overreach in American history. Imagine that it's the beginning of 2020 and you gave governors and health experts a report on an upcoming virus spread with the following parameters:

- It's most threatening to only the very elderly and those with specific underlying conditions (an identifiable segment of the population).
- The overall deaths in America would be within 2% of expected deaths for the year.
- The infection mortality rate would be 0.03%.

Then you ask: "Will you lock down your states? It may prompt the worst unemployment in nearly a century, shut down the healthcare system and education and fracture society." What do you think they would say? They wouldn't speak first. They would laugh. The early data well before the lockdowns, the data during the height of the April hospitalizations and the data in May and June all pointed to that.

The media perpetuated fear into the general populace, which drove polls supporting the lockdown and politicians buckled to those polls. Not all politicians, but most.

Suggested actions before ever locking down America again should include something like this:

- If we know the source (Wuhan in this case) and the host country is not forthcoming with information, invade it (February 2020 in this case) with a team of military and medical experts to ascertain for themselves the contagious spread probability. Then detail a profile of those susceptible to death, international protocols be damned. If they resist, embargo the whole country with the military. Leave the WHO out of it and go outside the CDC leadership for expertise. Sound extreme? So is locking down 300 million Americans for months and forcing 40 million into unemployment.

- A pandemic worthy of shutting down society must prove to be vulnerable to multiple segments of the population with no hope of controlling it. That was not the case here. An identifiable group was at risk and they could have been largely insulated.

When we see any story like this, we all need to research facts ourselves. We need to be independent thinkers. We cannot just blindly follow without exercising judgment. That's what America is. Early on, in March, friends told me the world would never be the same, but it would.

Five months into the pandemic in America, many actions were taken, some were excellent and some were fatal decisions. We made some drastic decisions affecting hundreds of millions of people from healthcare to schooling, employment to protection for the most vulnerable. How did the major actions perform, and how did other decisions made fare?

Action: Halting air travel between the United States and China
Grade: A
At the time the President halted air travel with China, all we knew was that a pandemic was spreading in China and it was bad enough for China to lockdown millions of their own people. This move would attempt to avoid a spread in America, a good call at the time with what we knew, as well as looking back.

Action: Declaring a national emergency
Grade: A
By declaring a national emergency, it enables quicker federal disaster relief to states. If a state follows by declaring a state of emergency, the normal (long) legislative time it takes to gets things done is circumvented, and relief can happen quickly, like was done with disaster relief efforts when Hurricane Katrina sunk New Orleans.

Action: February 27, Surgeon General Jerome Adams urging people not to wear masks because they do not prevent the transmission of SARS-CoV-2.
Grade: A
All the known science at the time was that cloth and paper masks do not prevent

the spread of airborne particles and pathogens. The surgeon general was right in calling that out, as did Dr. Tony Fauci in March.

Action: Halting air travel between the United States and Europe
Grade: A
Like the China travel ban, this was met with criticism, but in the moment, Europe was in a state of emergency in many countries, and with much unknown, this was a bold move.

Action: Federal government employs the Defense Production Act
Grade: B
This enabled the government to call on the private sector to produce what was needed in the interest of national security, or health in this case. However, pushing GM to manufacture ventilators and that whole frantic push when we were never really near capacity was a waste. Still, better safe than sorry.

Action: CDC report shows people of all ages at risk, March 18
Grade: F
It just wasn't true. While data from China was unreliable, early data from the cruise ships to Italy and other European countries showed that more than 90% of the deaths were to people with one or more pre-existing conditions, and in the absence of that, nearly all victims were over 70 with a median age over 80. COVID-19 was never life-threatening to all segments of the population. The CDC did a poor job throughout of explaining the difference between cases and those at risk and narrowing the scope of preventive efforts. Early on or not, the data was out there and the CDC was reckless in that message.

Action: Imperial College Model predicting up to 2.2MM deaths to COVID-19 in America
Grade: F
The model grossly overstated the COVID-19 fatality rates and predictive deaths and was simply illogical given the data we knew by early March. The author had a track record of predicting Spanish Flu-levels of impacts for previous pandemics, or potential pandemics. Then the author of the model would be caught violating the very stay-at-home order he started, while infected with COVID-19, to meet his married lover. You just can't make this stuff up.

Action: The Institute for Health Metrics and Evaluation (IHME) Models
Grade: F

Even after grossly overstating early predictions, the models would lose all reasonable credibility when they published updated models that would not be even near actual data the very day they were released.

Action: Cancelling college campus classes and moving to online
Grade: B

In the moment classes were cancelled, we did know the virus spread person-to-person and most college campuses are densely populated. The data never supported college age students at risk, but it's possible support staff may have been. Plus, college students had an online option so the overall effect to them was minimal compared to most.

Action: NCAA cancelling their tournament
Grade: B

The tournament should have been played without fans if the television revenue supported that.

Action: California leading the states with a ubiquitous lockdown
Grade: D

With no data supporting a fatality risk to all segments of the population, and data supporting just the opposite, Governor Newsom locked down his state. The media embraced it, Illinois followed, and the race was on. More than five million people lost their jobs, 40 million their liberties, and California would be one of the least affected states during the lockdown period, realizing a below average number of total deaths for 2020 into June, while renewing their lockdowns through the summer. Time for a leadership change.

Action: South Dakota not locking down
Grade: A

Governor Kristi Noem was the smartest governor in the room during the spring of 2020, and the boldest. No-Lockdown-Noem doesn't look it, but she may just have some Swedish blood in her after all. Governor Noem later committed to opening schools as normal in the fall of 2020, showing she really understands the data. Meanwhile, 11/15 largest school districts in America committed to going online in the fall.

Action: The Rolling Stones canceling their spring tour, March 17
Grade: A
With close fan contact in the audience, and the average age of the band over 75, this was a good move for them and their fans. I would miss out on seeing the band for the sixteenth and final time.

Action: CARES Act, March 27
Grade: A
This grade isn't giving an A for each piece of it, but with the government shutting the economy down, something had to give or there would have been a complete collapse of society all within a two-week period.

Action: CDC recommending face masks, April 3
Grade: C
It's a C because it would go too far and further justifications would not be outlined. Face masks in environments where social distancing was being practiced is ridiculous. The virus wasn't spreading outdoors like spring pollen. It was spreading within families that were locked down and nursing homes in the high majority of all hospitalizations. Recommending face masks outdoors in May and beyond would result in an F grade.

Action: Michigan protests in April and May
Grade: A
The first protest was a worthy demonstration against the lockdown policies, which prevented Michiganders from buying paint or garden supplies. And, any protest is a healthy expression regardless of where you land on the issue.

Action: Illinois leadership violating their own stay-at-home rules
Grade: F
If you're going to institute one of the toughest lockdowns in the country, you have to lead by example. Which means the mayor of Chicago shouldn't go get her hair done when no one else can, and the governor's wife shouldn't be leaving town to stay at their $12MM home in Florida. In a vacuum, those actions were completely fine, but they should have been fine for everyone or no one.

Action: Georgia announcing they would reopen April 24
Grade: A
Georgia was the first state to announce getting back to normal. Texas and Florida

and dozens more would follow their lead within days. Someone had to go first, an A for Governor Kemp. Georgia would continue to drop in cases, hospitalizations and deaths well after they reopened. Big surprise.

Action: Michigan, Illinois, California and others extending their lockdowns into June
Grade: F
Why? By May 1 it was very clear who was vulnerable, and rather than pour all efforts into protecting them, they extended blanketed shutdown orders that had minimal impact on hospitalizations (which were empty), and the economy was in ruins.

Action: Pre-K to 12 schools remaining closed for the 2019-2020 school year
Grade: F
Closing them early on is understandable. Not reopening them is unforgiveable. By as soon as mid-April, there was no data to support kids or healthy teachers/staff were at risk. Kids regressed, were locked down in their homes and like we saw in Wisconsin, parents vilified for play dates. This demonstrated a lack of the bold decision making that it took to shut them down in the first place, or just plain stubbornness.

Action: Texas reopening on May 1, albeit limited
Grade: A
Texas was pivotal in the reopening phase because it is, like California, an influential state because of its large population and economy. Only Texas of the very large states was bold enough to reopen in the face of data that was begging for this. Florida soon followed.

Action: Shelley Luther opening her salon in Dallas
Grade: A
With half of the COVID-19 deaths coming from nursing homes and care facilities in Texas, and Texas being one of the lowest per capita fatality states in the country, Texans needed to get back to work. In Luther's case, the first one through the wall is the bloodiest, but someone had to go first.

Action: Alex Berenson's Tweets
Grade: A
Berenson garnered national attention as the voice of data and reason throughout the lockdowns, with appearances on cable news, print media and his own podcasts. Berenson was the smartest guy in the room in the spring of 2020.

Action: Nursing home and long-term-care facility protections
Grade: F
Data was available early on from Italy that nursing homes were a hotbed for the spread and those residents were most vulnerable. It was known in America by mid-March. Few early policies were targeted to protect them and, in fact, policies did just the opposite. It took until May for the mainstream media to begin highlighting that deficiency and their vulnerability. More than half of all American COVID-19 deaths were sourced from nursing homes.

Action: The media
Grade: F
The media instilled fear into Americans that drove polls reflecting their support for continued lockdowns that drove politicians to keep people at home. The media never contextualized the cases rising with hospitalizations dropping (a good thing) and deaths decreasing (a great thing). The media had the lowest approval rating throughout the crisis.

Action: Lack of commitment to open schools as normal in the Fall 2020
Grade: F
There couldn't have been more data supporting that kids are not measurably affected by SARS-CoV-2 nor transmitters. Leaders in Canada and western Europe committed to open schools normally in the fall, yet in America the media, health officials and the government were noncommittal. Why?

Action: June 18, California requires "face coverings" in public
Grade: F
Only respirator/N95 face masks are effective at blocking airborne particles and pathogens. SARS-CoV-2 doesn't spread in the open air and hospitals were far from full of COVID-19 patients. People wearing cloth or non-respirator face coverings may be worse off than wearing nothing. One more demonstration that leaders didn't understand the data. Weeks later "cases" rose sharply in California, demonstrating face masks did not impact the virus being the virus. It just had to run its course.

Action: June 26, stalled reopening's and more lockdowns in Texas and Florida
Grade: F
Cases were "surging", yet COVID-19 hospitalizations were not, and fatalities were

no higher than April. The United States was at 20% the fatalities from the April peak even with backdated additions, and in those states COVID-19 fatalities were 5% of their daily total. Where could we get a Biology 101 or Statistics 101 student to begin leading this effort?

Action: CDC Director Robert Redfield calling out in July that the health risks of keeping schools closed are greater than those of opening them
Grade: A
With kids at virtually no measurable risk of catching nor transmitting COVID-19, and most other countries committing to reopen schools as normal in the fall, this was an important message for our kids and education.

Action: Mid-July, CDC counting of provisional deaths, which is all-cause mortality
Grade: D
We've discussed all-cause mortality as the most reliable data point. In mid-July, all-cause mortality went up from 102% to 108% in a couple days, and we went from 35/50 states flat or below average to 11/50 states. Something worth questioning happened with the data just as some in the media and me were calling out the low all-cause impact we'd been seeing. Deaths from weeks and even months prior were counted as current COVID-19 deaths.

Action: Media reporting on Florida "surge"
Grade: F
In July 150,000 new "cases" were reported in Florida in a two-week period while hospitalizations, ICU usage and deaths stayed flat. That's a huge success story that was never reported by the media. Why?

Action: State-wide "face covering" order in Texas in July
Grade: F
It became comical, people wearing dirty bandanas over their face, paper or thin fabric masks that could not offer any protection against a potential spread of a virus, just to comply with the state order. In one hilarious case, two guys walked in Subway, one with his shirt over his face and the other with an empty McDonald's cup around his nose and mouth so they could get served.

Action: July 2, guy walking alone down my street on a sunny one hundred-degree Dallas day, wearing a facemask
Grade: N/A
As he walked down my street, I felt sad for him. If only he knew the data....

CHAPTER 22

JUNE 30, 2020

I began writing this book on April 6, 2020 and finished the first draft 25 days later. Most of May was spent updating and cleaning it up. Most of June was spent getting it self-published. In an effort to get the information out timely, I did not secure a major publisher like my past books. That process is a lengthy one.

As you lived this and know, the information changes fast and daily. COVID-19 activity lightened up significantly in May. States that reopened remained "flat" for several weeks. Hospitals opened up to non-COVID-19 procedures. Testing accelerated. As those things happened, cases rose in June. They spiked most in Florida, Texas and Arizona, hot summer states. Where we may have thought that like other respiratory viruses, activity would cool in the heat, it did not.

Texas cases went up in late June five to ten times what they were when New York was getting the brunt of activity in March and April. Florida's went up five-fold. Arizona was up close to ten-fold. The media was reporting again like they did in March and April.

More importantly, getting accurate data was very difficult. As "cases" grew, which we know are positive tests of the virus, antibodies, or COVID-19 itself, meaning symptomatic, what was really happening? All we knew for certain at the end of June was cases were up and lockdowns were back, or reopening's stalled.

The data will continue to unfold into 2020 and beyond. As you consider the headlines, we all need to know the following things to evaluate for ourselves what is happening and the severity of it all:

1. If cases are up, exactly what are the demographics of the cases? This includes age, pre-existing conditions, etc.

2. How many "cases" are asymptomatic and how many are symptomatic and then hospitalized?
3. How many reach the ICU?
4. What is the COVID-19-related ICU usage compared to capacity? What was the capacity a year ago?
5. Did the patient get hospitalized from COVID-19 or with SARS-CoV-2?
6. If the victim died, was it directly from a COVID-19 prompted condition or something else?
7. We're told to wear face masks. How does a non-respirator type of mask help? How exactly does SARS-CoV-2 spread outdoors in the open air? Hint: it doesn't and they don't.
8. What is the context of COVID-19 deaths? While the media admonished Texas and Florida for reopening, their COVID-19-coded deaths in June were about 5% of the average daily deaths in those states.
9. With the loose coding of COVID-19 hospitalizations and fatalities, what is the actual all-cause death data? Is it up or down to our averages, and by a significant amount either way? That's how we know the real COVID-19 impact.

Ask these questions. Demand answers. This is not a political book or analysis. The health experts and media have failed us in this challenging time, and those failures have driven policies. Is it a media thirst for dirty laundry or do they just not understand the data, contextualize it for us? In late June, a writer for the *Washington Post* hypothesized that Fox News reporting caused a spike in cases. Help us all.

As cases grew in those three southern states, COVID-19 fatalities stayed fairly stable to what they were in the spring. Cases rose much more than hospitalizations and deaths. The average age of positive tests was younger in June. Most were asymptomatic. What this means is the analysis in the middle of this book, and dating back to the cruise ships, is holding. Still, getting timely answers to these questions is ridiculously difficult.

The CDC estimated in June that ten times the reported "cases" are probably in existence in America. My opinion? If you drew a line between our official 2.5MM cases and 100MM, it's closer to the latter. The random samplings discussed earlier suggest that, as well as the huge increase in "cases." The quest here is for accurate data and reasonable conclusions drawn based on that data. At the end of June Dr. Fauci stated with a doomsday tone that the United States may experience 100,000 cases a day. No kidding.

What he should have said was *"We may uncover 100,000 more people per day in the United States that have had exposure to SARS-CoV-2 or COVID-19. At the rate we're going, with cases up and hospitalizations and deaths down, this is looking less dangerous than we thought. This is good news!"*

Below are the charts of both cases and deaths in the United States through June 30, 2020. Do you see anything insightful?

Daily New Cases

Cases per Day
Data as of 0:00 GMT+0

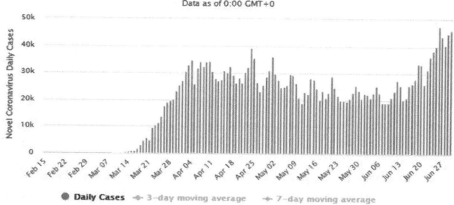

Source: https://www.worldometers.info/coronavirus/country/us

Daily Deaths

Deaths per Day
Data as of 0:00 GMT+8

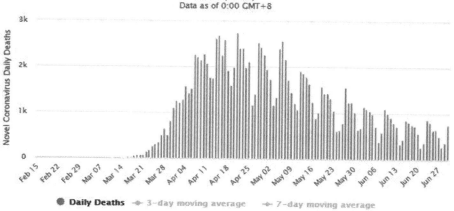

Source: https://www.worldometers.info/coronavirus/country/us

"Cases" *are* surging. Hospitalizations are spiked some but not like we saw in the spring. Deaths are moving in the other direction, and the latter includes backdated and probable COVID-19 deaths as of June 26 when counting changed. It also includes many deaths *with* SARS-CoV-2, not *from* COVID-19. This is weeks after the congregations surrounding the George Floyd protests, states reopening, people easing into some kind of normal. Still, we keep being told, "Wait two more weeks!"

It's becoming depressing as small businesses are permanently closed now. Thousands of restaurants will never reopen. Overdoses are skyrocketing. Unmaintained health conditions are filling up hospitals more than COVID-19. New York City, between the lockdowns and the protests, will take years to recover. Schools are threatening to go online; 11/15 of the largest school districts indicated they are going online in the fall. The service industry is a long way from recovery.

FACE COVERINGS

Face coverings are mandated in many cities and states now. Do they help? Does a non-respirator, cloth of any kind face covering do anything? It's an interesting analysis. Prior to 2020, there is a plethora of data out there that stated that cloth face coverings do not provide protection against airborne particles and pathogens – a virus. Still, the media and politicians are mandating it all over.

Here is some pre-COVID-19 analysis on the benefits of cloth face coverings. In 2017 *The Lancet* featured an article called "Clearing the air: do facemasks protect health?"[325] In it they stated:

Traditional facemasks can be made of paper or cloth (originally cotton gauze), and they provide a physical barrier between the mouth and nose and the outside environment. These include the traditional surgical masks associated with doctors and dentists, which are made of paper or other non-woven materials. They can protect the wearer from potentially harmful substances (eg, blood spray); however, they do not provide protection from airborne particles or pathogens.

A 2017 Oxford Academic article[326] offered this on face masks:

With one exception case-control studies consistently reported a protective effect of medical N95 masks against SARS. Compared to no rPPE" controls, N95 respirators conferred protection against confirmed SARS-CoV infection in 2 of 3 case-control studies. No protective effect against SARS was reported for disposable cotton or paper masks.

In 2020 Dr. Denis G. Rancourt authored this analysis[327] on the value of face masks in protecting people from SARS-CoV-2:

By making mask-wearing recommendations and policies for the general public, or by expressly condoning the practice, governments have both ignored the scientific evidence and done the opposite of following the precautionary principle. In an absence of knowledge, governments should not make policies that have a hypothetical potential to cause harm. The government has an onus barrier before it instigates a broad social-engineering intervention, or allows corporations to exploit fear-based sentiments. Furthermore, individuals should know that there is no known benefit arising from wearing a mask in a viral respiratory illness epidemic, and that scientific studies have shown that any benefit must be residually small, compared to other and determinative factors.

By far the most interesting piece I found was a very detailed analysis published in 2016 by the Oral Health Group.[328] The article is now redacted as of 2020, as seen below:

Feature

Update: Why Face Masks Don't Work: A Revealing Review

October 18, 2016
by Oral Health

If you are looking for "Why Face Masks Don't Work: A Revealing Review" by John Hardie, BDS, MSc, PhD, FRCDC, it has been removed. The content was published in 2016 and is no longer relevant in our current climate.

Please note that the content from Oral Health Group is primarily intended to educate and inform dental professionals.

However, in the original article, which you can find in the archives footnoted, they made the following assertions based on their analysis:

Traditionally face masks have been recommended to protect the mouth and nose from the "droplet" route of infection, presumably because they will prevent the inhalation of relatively large particles. Their efficacy must be re-examined in light of the fact that aerosols contain particles many times smaller than 5 microns. Prior to this examination, it is pertinent to review the defense mechanism of the respiratory tract.

No matter how well a mask conforms to the shape of a person's face, it is not designed to create an airtight seal around the face. Masks will always fit fairly loosely with considerable gaps along the cheeks, around the bridge of the nose and along the bottom edge of the mask below the chin. These gaps do not provide adequate protection as they permit the passage of air and aerosols when the wearer inhales. It is important to appreciate that if masks contained filters capable of trapping viruses, the peripheral gaps around the masks would continue to permit the inhalation of unfiltered air and aerosols.

It should be no surprise that a study of eight brands of face masks found that they did not filter out 20-100% of particles varying in size from 0.1 to 4.0 microns. Another investigation showed penetration ranges from 5-100% when masks were challenged with relatively large 1.0 micron particles. A further study found that masks were incapable of filtering out 80-85% of particles varying in size from 0.3 to 2.0 microns.

The filter material of surgical masks does not retain or filter out submicron particles; surgical masks are not designed to eliminate air leakage around the edges; surgical masks do not protect the wearer from inhaling small particles that can remain airborne for long periods of time.

The complete article is very lengthy and cited with 36 reputable sources by medical journal standards. Why was the analysis good enough for the Oral Health Group to publish and support four years ago but not now? Did the science behind a virus and non-respirator mask change? If so, where was their credibility then? We can all visit indoor shopping areas and see the variation of masks people are wearing? Does the CDC, Dr. Fauci, anyone credible actually believe that a "face covering" that may well be a bandana pulled up over the user's mouth and nose prevent the spread of fine particles like SARS-CoV-2?

This isn't about one being anti-masks. There's a complete consensus that driving while intoxicated is unsafe. Engaging in unprotected sex while HIV positive is unsafe. The list is long of accepted practices we should all endure to keep each other safe. Prior to the summer of 2020, there was no acceptance that "face coverings" protect users or others from a virus. In February 2020, the surgeon general Jerome Adams said, *"Seriously people — STOP BUYING MASKS! They are NOT effective in preventing general public from catching #Coronavirus."*[329] Did science change in five months? Virus transmission certainly could not have changed.

We have plenty of data in front of us to suggest it's time to get back to normal. At this point Americans are perfectly able to judge for themselves whether they want to go out or not. States should reopen and businesses and entertainment venues can require indemnity releases from their customers, creating a freedom of choice. State and local leaders are governing as if they are pulling puppet strings on businesses, on taxpayers, on citizens. The data just doesn't support their orders.

The case is laid out against the lockdowns. What is your verdict?

Share your feedback with me. You may agree with this analysis and you may not. I'm open to learning from you. I'd like to hear from you, your thoughts and experiences. I hope to share those in *After the Lockdowns*. I hope we get there soon.

Michael
michaelgbetrus@gmail.com

ENDNOTES

1   Merriam Webster Dictionary
2   https://www.who.int/gho/hiv/en/
3   https://www.kshs.org/kansapedia/flu-epidemic-of-1918/17805
4   https://www.nationalgeographic.com/news/2014/1/140123-spanish-flu-1918-china-origins-pandemic-science-health/
5   https://www.cdc.gov/flu/pandemic-resources/1918-pandemic-h1n1.html
6   US Department of Health, Education, and Welfare 1956.
7   https://www.ecohealthalliance.org/2018/05/outbreak-pandemic-strikes?gclid=Cj0KCQjw-Mr0BRDyARIsAKEFbeey1pvEww3GFeOyIVvhWFo9eAZdp3OS1iDiJuGlXhSjySZp9cZwJxAaApdDEALw_wcB
8   https://www.history.com/news/spanish-flu-pandemic-response-cities
9   https://www.cdc.gov/nchs/pressroom/sosmap/flu_pneumonia_mortality/flu_pneumonia.htm
10 https://www.thelancet.com/journals/lancet/article/PIIS0140-6736(03)15329-9/fulltext
11 https://www.deccanchronicle.com/world/asia/060520/what-happens-at-the-wuhan-institute-of-virology.html
12 https://www.thelancet.com/journals/lancet/article/PIIS0140-6736(20)30183-5/fulltext
13 https://www.indexmundi.com/iran/age_structure.html
14 https://thefederalist.com/2020/03/17/iran-and-italy-are-paying-a-hefty-price-for-close-ties-with-communist-china/
15 https://www.rnz.co.nz/news/national/408675/nz-to-close-doors-on-foreign-travellers-from-china
16 https://www.cnn.com/2020/02/07/health/coronavirus-travel-ban/index.html
17 https://thehill.com/homenews/campaign/481028-biden-slams-trump-for-cutting-health-programs-before-coronavirus-outbreak

18   https://www.bls.gov/opub/ted/2020/unemployment-rate-2-percent-for-college-grads-3-8-percent-for-high-school-grads-in-january-2020.htm

19   https://www.denverpost.com/2020/01/24/colorado-unemployment-rate-historic-low/

20   https://www.sltrib.com/news/politics/2020/01/24/utahs-unemployment-rate/

21   https://www.cnbc.com/2020/01/23/weekly-jobless-claims.html

22   https://www.orlandoweekly.com/Blogs/archives/2020/01/24/floridas-unemployment-rate-hits-record-low-but-how-does-orlando-rank

23   https://www.marketwatch.com/story/new-jobless-claims-fall-5th-straight-week-to-204000-in-sign-of-strong-us-labor-market-2020-01-16

24   https://mynorthwest.com/1680642/washington-unemployment-rate-2019/

25   https://www.crainsdetroit.com/economy/michigan-unemployment-down-payroll-jobs-advanced-throughout-2019

26   https://www.edd.ca.gov/newsroom/unemployment-january-2020.htm

27   https://www.fox10phoenix.com/news/dow-closes-above-29000-for-the-first-time

28   https://www.wsj.com/articles/rank-and-file-workers-get-bigger-raises-11577442600

29   https://www.nytimes.com/2020/02/03/nyregion/nyc-coronavirus-what-we-know.html

30   https://www.cbsnews.com/news/transcript-dr-anthony-fauci-on-face-the-nation-february-16-2020/

31   https://www.nytimes.com/2020/02/24/us/politics/trump-coronavirus-response.html

32   https://www.bloomberg.com/news/articles/2020-02-06/coronavirus-places-that-have-placed-china-travel-restrictions

33   https://www.cnbc.com/2020/02/17/coronavirus-could-impact-5-million-companies-worldwide-research-shows.html

34   https://www.sourcify.com/the-top-10-products-manufactured-in-china-in-2018/

35   Trendforce 2020

36   https://www.econlib.org/great-moments-in-epidemiology/

37   https://cmmid.github.io/topics/covid19/diamond_cruise_cfr_estimates.html

38   https://www.bbc.com/news/world-asia-51568496

39   https://www.thelancet.com/journals/laninf/article/PIIS1473-3099(20)30244-9/fulltext)

40   https://www.theguardian.com/world/2020/mar/13/from-paradise-to-coronavirus-the-grand-princess-and-the-cruise-from-hell

41   https://www.theguardian.com/world/2020/mar/13/from-paradise-to-coronavirus-the-grand-princess-and-the-cruise-from-hell

42   https://www.cdc.gov/mmwr/volumes/69/wr/mm6912e3.htm

43   https://www.cnbc.com/2020/04/13/navy-sailor-of-roosevelt-carrier-dies-from-coronavirus.html

ENDNOTES

44 https://www.aljazeera.com/news/2020/04/660-french-aircraft-carrier-crew-infected-coronavirus-200415191827292.html

45 https://www.topuniversities.com/universities/imperial-college-london

46 https://www.usnews.com/education/best-global-universities/imperial-college-london-505571

47 https://pubmed.ncbi.nlm.nih.gov/19628172/

48 https://www.theguardian.com/world/2005/sep/30/birdflu.jamessturcke

49 https://www.theguardian.com/world/2005/sep/30/birdflu.jamessturcke

50 https://www.theguardian.com/education/2002/jan/09/research.highereducation

51 https://www.imperial.ac.uk/news/196234/covid-19-imperial-researchers-model-likely-impact/

52 https://www.imperial.ac.uk/media/imperial-college/medicine/sph/ide/gida-fellowships/Imperial-College-COVID19-NPI-modelling-16-03-2020.pdf

53 https://www.telegraph.co.uk/technology/2020/05/16/coding-led-lockdown-totally-unreliable-buggy-mess-say-experts/

54 https://www.aha.org/statistics/fast-facts-us-hospitals

55 https://www.telegraph.co.uk/news/2020/04/04/science-clash-imperial-vs-oxford-sex-smear-created-rival-covid/

56 https://www.usnews.com/news/health-news/articles/2020-03-30/odds-of-hospitalization-death-with-covid-19-rise-steadily-with-age-study

57 https://www.telegraph.co.uk/news/2020/06/02/prof-lockdown-neil-ferguson-admits-sweden-used-science-uk-has/

58 https://www.telegraph.co.uk/news/2020/04/04/science-clash-imperial-vs-oxford-sex-smear-created-rival-covid/

59 https://www.newscientist.com/article/2238578-uk-has-enough-intensive-care-units-for-coronavirus-expert-predicts/

60 https://www.washingtonexaminer.com/news/is-the-coronavirus-as-deadly-as-they-say-professors-claim-more-data-needed-to-know-mortality-rate

61 https://www.washingtonpost.com/health/2020/04/06/americas-most-influential-coronavirus-model-just-revised-its-estimates-downward-not-every-model-agrees/

62 https://www.medrxiv.org/content/10.1101/2020.03.27.20043752v1.full.pdf

63 https://www.rochesterfirst.com/news/state-news/watch-live-gov-cuomos-daily-briefing-amid-covid-19-outbreak-in-new-york-state-4/

64 https://www.nytimes.com/2020/04/01/us/la-county-coronavirus-hospitals.html

65 https://www1.nyc.gov/site/doh/covid/covid-19-data.page

66 https://nypost.com/2020/03/19/new-york-coronavirus-cases-reach-2959-with-8000-tests-conducted-overnight/

67   https://hcpresources.medtronic.com/blog/high-acuity-ventilator-cost-guide

68   https://www1.nyc.gov/site/doh/covid/covid-19-data.page

69   https://www.silive.com/coronavirus/2020/04/coronavirus-state-issues-list-of-3565-deaths-by-age.html

70   https://www.medrxiv.org/content/10.1101/2020.04.08.20057794v1

71   https://obesity.procon.org/global-obesity-levels/

72   https://morningconsult.com/governor-rankings/

73   https://www.nytimes.com/2020/02/06/nyregion/bill-de-blasio-mayor-nyc.html

74   https://www.politico.com/states/new-york/albany/story/2020/03/28/de-blasios-coronavirus-crisis-1269480

75   https://scri.siena.edu/2020/03/30/87-of-nyers-approve-of-cuomos-handling-of-the-coronavirus/

76   https://www.nytimes.com/2020/03/30/us/politics/andrew-cuomo.html

77   https://www.theguardian.com/us-news/2020/apr/04/andrew-cuomo-profile-coronavirus-new-york

78   https://credder.com/article/15640/bloomberg-are-you-a-robot-34162074-f39c-40c5-866b-2b29ec126a7e

79   https://www.washingtontimes.com/news/2020/apr/8/inside-the-beltway-andrew-cuomo-frenzy-builds-in-a/

80   https://www.washingtontimes.com/news/2020/apr/8/inside-the-beltway-andrew-cuomo-frenzy-builds-in-a/

81   https://www.washingtontimes.com/news/2020/apr/8/inside-the-beltway-andrew-cuomo-frenzy-builds-in-a/

82   https://www.washingtontimes.com/news/2020/apr/8/inside-the-beltway-andrew-cuomo-frenzy-builds-in-a/

83   https://twitter.com/NYCMayor/status/1255309615883063297?s=20

84   https://www.independent.co.uk/news/health/coronavirus-italy-hospitals-doctor-lockdown-quarantine-intensive-care-a9401186.html

85   https://www.ons.gov.uk/peoplepopulationandcommunity/healthandsocialcare/conditionsanddiseases/articles/coronaviruscovid19roundup/2020-03-26

86   https://www.manilatimes.net/2020/06/06/opinion/columnists/topanalysis/swedens-covid-strategist-owns-mistakes-norway-wishes-it-had-acted-more-like-sweden/729711/

87   https://verfassungsblog.de/icelands-rule-of-common-sense-and-law/

88   https://www.nytimes.com/2020/03/24/world/asia/india-coronavirus-lockdown.html

89   https://travel.state.gov/content/travel/en/international-travel.html

90   https://calmatters.org/health/coronavirus/2020/04/california-coronavirus-covid-patient-hospitalization-data-icu/

91   https://kesq.com/news/2020/04/10/riverside-county-unveils-app-to-report-coronavirus-violations/

92   https://covid19.alabama.gov/#live-updates

93   http://dhss.alaska.gov/dph/Epi/id/Pages/COVID-19/default.aspx

94   https://azdhs.gov/preparedness/epidemiology-disease-control/infectious-disease-epidemiology/covid-19/dashboards/index.php

95   https://www.healthy.arkansas.gov/programs-services/topics/novel-coronavirus

96   https://www.modernhealthcare.com/hospitals/covid-19-could-fill-hospital-beds-how-many-are-there

97   https://www.modernhealthcare.com/hospitals/covid-19-could-fill-hospital-beds-how-many-are-there

98   https://portal.ct.gov/-/media/Coronavirus/CTDPHCOVID19summary4212020.pdf?la=en

99   https://www.tcpalm.com/story/news/2020/04/22/coronavirus-florida-confirmed-cases-deaths-hospitalizations/3002095001/

100   https://dph.georgia.gov/covid-19-daily-status-report

101   https://health.hawaii.gov/coronavirusdisease2019/

102   https://dph.illinois.gov/covid19/hospitalization-utilization

103   https://coronavirus.iowa.gov/

104   https://www.kansas.com/news/coronavirus/article242469771.html#adnrb=900000

105   https://covidtracking.com/data

106   http://ldh.la.gov/Coronavirus/

107   https://www.pressherald.com/2020/04/28/maine-cdc-reports-17-additional-coronavirus-cases-but-no-new-deaths/#

108   https://www.pressherald.com/2020/04/18/hospitalizations-in-much-of-maine-have-flattened-or-decreased-over-past-week/#

109   https://coronavirus.maryland.gov/

110   https://www.mass.gov/doc/covid-19-dashboard-may-7-2020/download

111   https://www.clickondetroit.com/health/2020/04/09/michigan-offers-new-hospital-data-on-coronavirus-patients-medical-supplies/

112   https://www.michigan.gov/coronavirus/0,9753,7-406-98163-520743--,00.html

113   https://www.metrotimes.com/detroit/why-did-michigan-get-hit-by-the-coronavirus-harder-than-its-neighbors/Content?oid=24382884

114   https://www.washingtonpost.com/outlook/2020/03/25/hydroxychloroquine-false-hope-trump/

115   https://www.michigan.gov/documents/lara/Reminder_of_Appropriate_Prescribing_and_Dispensing_3-24-2020_684869_7.pdf

116 https://www.nytimes.com/2020/04/01/health/hydroxychloroquine-coronavirus-malaria.html

117 https://nypost.com/2020/04/02/hydroxychloroquine-most-effective-coronavirus-treatment-poll/

118 https://www.nationalreview.com/news/detroit-dems-to-censure-state-lawmaker-who-thanked-trump-for-touting-chloroquine/

119 https://www.detroitnews.com/story/news/local/detroit-city/2020/04/25/detroit-democrats-unanimously-censure-lawmaker-karen-whitsett-who-credited-trump-covid-19-recovery/3025907001/

120 https://www.health.nd.gov/diseases-conditions/coronavirus/north-dakota-coronavirus-cases

121 https://coronavirus.ohio.gov/wps/portal/gov/covid-19/dashboards/overview

122 https://web.archive.org/web/20200425130930/https://www.health.pa.gov/topics/Documents/Diseases%20and%20Conditions/COVID-19%20Interim%20Nursing%20Facility%20Guidance.pdf

123 https://www.arcgis.com/apps/opsdashboard/index.html#/85054b06472e4208b02285b8557f24cf

124 https://ri-department-of-health-covid-19-data-rihealth.hub.arcgis.com/

125 https://scdhec.gov/infectious-diseases/viruses/coronavirus-disease-2019-covid-19/sc-testing-data-projections-covid-19

126 https://doh.sd.gov/news/coronavirus.aspx

127 https://txdshs.maps.arcgis.com/apps/opsdashboard/index.html#/ed483ecd702b4298ab01e8b9cafc8b83

128 https://www.deseret.com/utah/2020/4/2/21204511/coronavirus-why-doesnt-utah-have-stay-at-home-order-covid-19-salt-lake

129 https://coronavirus-dashboard.utah.gov/

130 https://www.doh.wa.gov/Portals/1/Documents/1600/coronavirus/data-tables/covid-hospital-summary.pdf

131 https://pjmedia.com/culture/megan-fox/2020/04/29/new-normal-wisconsin-cops-caught-on-camera-threatening-mom-for-letting-child-play-with-neighbor-n386692

132 https://www.dhs.wisconsin.gov/covid-19/cases.htm

133 https://medcitynews.com/2020/04/report-pathologist-says-abbotts-rapid-covid-19-test-produces-15-false-negative-rate/

134 https://drexel.edu/dornsife/news/latest-news/2020/May/how-many-lives-have-stay-at-home-orders-saved/

135 https://www.thebalance.com/dow-jones-closing-history-top-highs-and-lows-since-1929-3306174

ENDNOTES

136 https://www.cnn.com/world/live-news/coronavirus-outbreak-03-25-20-intl-hnk/index.html

137 HR 748—38 (SEC. 2104)

138 https://fileunemployment.org/unemployment-benefits/unemployment-benefits-comparison-by-state/

139 https://fileunemployment.org/unemployment-benefits/unemployment-benefits-comparison-by-state/

140 https://fred.stlouisfed.org/series/MEPAINUSA672N

141 https://www.vox.com/2020/3/25/21194278/lindsey-graham-coronavirus-stimulus

142 https://home.treasury.gov/policy-issues/cares/assistance-for-american-workers-and-families

143 a former Section Chief at the Board of Governors of the Federal Reserve System and a current policy director at the Washington Center for Equitable Growth (left side of the spectrum)

144 https://www.hamiltonproject.org/assets/files/Sahm_web_20190506.pdf (p. 70)

145 HR 748–280-283

146 https://www.voiceofsandiego.org/topics/news/san-diego-health-care-providers-are-bleeding-money/

147 HR 748–218 (SEC. 4112)

148 Sum of figures in HR 748–21-22 (SEC. 1107)

149 748–190 (SEC 4003)

150 https://www.cnbc.com/2020/04/21/coronavirus-senate-passes-484-billion-small-business-relief-bill.html

151 https://www.axios.com/trump-signs-interim-coronavirus-relief-bill-192d7b83-ec92-4fa9-9f8c-be241e886192.html

152 https://www.cnbc.com/2020/03/27/house-passes-2-trillion-coronavirus-stimulus-bill-sends-it-to-trump.html

153 https://thehill.com/homenews/senate/489470-mcconnell-says-2t-bill-is-emergency-relief-and-not-a-stimulus

154 https://www.denverpost.com/2020/03/27/trump-signs-coronavirus-stimulus/

155 https://www.bloomberg.com/news/articles/2020-03-27/trump-signs-2-trillion-virus-bill-largest-ever-u-s-stimulus

156 https://thehill.com/homenews/state-watch/489653-cuomo-calls-2t-stimulus-reckless-says-it-failed-to-meet-local-government

157 "It's Raining Cash," ep. 980 of The Ben Shapiro Show

158 https://www.realclearpolitics.com/video/2020/04/25/maher_to_pelosi_spending_funny_money_could_end_up_hurting_more_people_than_the_coronavirus.html

159 https://finance.yahoo.com/news/mark-cuban-on-paycheck-protection-program-for-

small-businesses-loans-234227330.html

160 https://newsradiowrva.radio.com/blogs/jeff-katz/mark-cuban-praises-trumps-handling-of-covid-19

161 https://www.cnbc.com/2020/03/15/federal-reserve-cuts-rates-to-zero-and-launches-massive-700-billion-quantitative-easing-program.html

162 https://www.foxbusiness.com/markets/us-stocks-april-20-2020

163 https://finance.yahoo.com/news/oil-prices-climb-storage-fills-013327734.html

164 https://blogs.edweek.org/edweek/campaign-k-12/2020/04/teacher_pension_plans_coronavirus.html

165 https://www.hotelmanagement.net/own/studies-break-down-covid-19-s-impact-hotels-travel-plans

166 https://www.galioninquirer.com/news/53328/survey-nearly-90-percent-of-small-businesses-negatively-impacted-by-coronavirus

167 https://www.npr.org/2020/04/09/829753752/small-town-hospitals-are-closing-just-as-coronavirus-arrives-in-rural-america

168 https://www.beckershospitalreview.com/finance/5-washington-hospitals-face-imminent-closure-as-covid-19-wreaks-havoc.html

169 https://www.beckershospitalreview.com/largest-hospitals-and-health-systems-in-america-2019.html

170 https://www.healthcaredive.com/news/healthcare-sector-lost-stunning-14m-jobs-in-april/577630/

171 https://www.washingtonpost.com/health/starved-for-cash-hospitals-and-doctor-groups-cut-staff-amid-pandemic/2020/04/09/d3593f54-79a7-11ea-a130-df573469f094_story.html

172 https://www.washingtontimes.com/news/2020/apr/28/merck-cuts-2020-forecasts-sees-big-pandemic-impact/

173 https://www.itv.com/news/2020-04-22/60-000-cancer-patients-could-die-because-of-lack-of-treatment-or-diagnosis-oncologist-on-coronavirus-dilemma/

174 https://www.fightcancer.org/releases/survey-covid-19-affecting-patients'-access-cancer-care

175 http://www.stoptb.org/assets/documents/news/Modeling%20Report_1%20May%202020_FINAL.pdfon

176 https://www.washingtonpost.com/nation/2020/06/01/americans-are-delaying-medical-care-its-devastating-health-care-providers/?arc404=true

177 https://www.washingtonpost.com/business/2020/04/21/netflix-adds-whopping-16-million-subscribers-worldwide-coronavirus-keeps-people-home/

178 https://www.foxbusiness.com/markets/coronavirus-pandemic-amazon-technology-

headaches-bezos

179 https://www.cdc.gov/nchs/nvss/vsrr/COVID19/index.htm

180 https://www.cdc.gov/nchs/data/nvss/coronavirus/Alert-2-New-ICD-code-introduced-for-COVID-19-deaths.pdf

181 https://www.cdc.gov/coronavirus/2019-ncov/cases-updates/cases-in-us.html

182 https://www.nytimes.com/2020/04/14/nyregion/new-york-coronavirus-deaths.html

183 https://www.politico.com/states/new-york/albany/story/2020/04/14/new-york-city-coronavirus-death-toll-jumps-by-3-700-after-uncounted-fatalities-are-added-1275931

184 https://www.foxnews.com/media/physician-blasts-cdc-coronavirus-death-count-guidelines

185 https://revcycleintelligence.com/news/hospital-reimbursement-for-uninsured-covid-19-cases-may-total-42b

186 https://revcycleintelligence.com/news/hospitals-to-lose-1k-per-covid-19-case-despite-medicare-rate-bump

187 https://www.foxnews.com/us/pa-removes-200-deaths-official-coronavirus-count-questions-mount-reporting-process-data-accuracy

188 https://denver.cbslocal.com/2020/04/30/coronavirus-nursing-home-deaths-colorado-public-health/

189 https://durangoherald.com/articles/324539-montezuma-county-disputes-states-coronavirus-death-count

190 https://www.businessinsider.com/half-europes-covid-19-deaths-in-long-term-care-facilities-2020-4)

191 https://www.dispatch.com/news/20200521/70-of-ohio-coronavirus-deaths-have-occurred-in-long-term-care-facilities

192 https://www.nytimes.com/interactive/2020/05/09/us/coronavirus-cases-nursing-homes-us.html

193 https://www.sfchronicle.com/bayarea/article/Nearly-half-of-California-s-COVID-19-deaths-are-15258337.php

194 https://chicago.suntimes.com/coronavirus/2020/5/8/21252728/nursing-homes-coronavirus-deaths-illinois-48-percent-covid-19

195 www.kansascity.com › news › local › article242262076

196 https://www.wbur.org/commonhealth/2020/04/24/seniors-coronavirus-nursing-homes-testing

197 https://www.indystar.com/story/news/investigations/2020/04/27/nursing-homes-now-account-one-third-indiana-coronavirus-deaths/3034770001/

198 https://coloradosun.com/2020/04/22/colorado-nursing-home-deaths-rise-

coronavirus-covid19/

199 https://riverdalepress.com/stories/queens-bronx-lead-covid-nursing-home-deaths-coronavirus-nyc,71677

200 https://www.walb.com/2020/04/24/reports-georgias-covid-deaths-were-residents-long-term-care-facilities/

201 https://www.iberianet.com/news/coronavirus/nursing-home-resident-covid-19-deaths-continue-to-rise/article_88577500-7f44-11ea-8748-1fc173c19f04.html

202 https://www.washingtonpost.com/world/europe/nursing-homes-coronavirus-deaths-europe/2020/04/23/d635619c-8561-11ea-81a3-9690c9881111_story.html

203 https://wwmt.com/news/local/state-of-michigan-reports-more-than-2000-nursing-home-patients-have-covid-19

204 https://www.fox13news.com/news/outlook-for-covid-19-in-floridas-long-term-care-facilities-worsens-as-new-data-emerges

205 https://nypost.com/2020/04/23/coronavirus-deaths-at-us-nursing-homes-reach-over-10000/

206 https://www.thecentersquare.com/virginia/nearly-60-percent-of-virginia-s-coronavirus-deaths-are-in-nursing-homes-other-long-term/article_3c9d1152-94a6-11ea-b37b-bb1588c0d0bf.html

207 https://www.expressnews.com/news/local/article/40-percent-of-coronavirus-deaths-in-Texas-linked-15238887.php

208 https://www.mcall.com/coronavirus/mc-nws-pa-transparency-virus-wolf-20200506-dqmz7wbhtnalhhj7rne2r5cmru-story.html

209 https://www.startribune.com/minn-nursing-homes-already-site-of-81-of-covid-19-deaths-still-taking-in-infected-patients/570601282/

210 https://www.newsweek.com/deaths-coronavirus-are-devastating-nursing-homes-united-states-1502408

211 https://www.washingtonpost.com/world/the_americas/coronavirus-canada-long-term-care-nursing-homes/2020/05/18/01494ad4-947f-11ea-87a3-22d324235636_story.html

212 https://www.nytimes.com/2020/04/24/us/nursing-homes-coronavirus.html

213 https://ltccovid.org/wp-content/uploads/2020/05/Mortality-associated-with-COVID-3-May-final-6.pdf

214 https://ltccovid.org/wp-content/uploads/2020/05/Mortality-associated-with-COVID-3-May-final-6.pdf

215 https://www.medrxiv.org/content/10.1101/2020.04.28.20083147v1.full.pdf

216 https://www.cdc.gov/nchs/nvss/vsrr/covid19/index.htm

217 https://www.mdch.state.mi.us/osr/Provisional/MontlyDxCounts.asp#

218   https://www.sciencedirect.com/science/article/pii/S1201971219303285

219   https://www.reuters.com/article/us-health-coronavirus-new-orleans/why-is-new-orleans-coronavirus-death-rate-twice-new-yorks-obesity-is-a-factor-idUSKBN21K1B0

220   https://www.sciencenews.org/article/coronavirus-covid19-obesity-risk-factor

221   https://www.washingtonpost.com/health/2020/04/24/strokes-coronavirus-young-patients/

222   https://www.cdc.gov/nchs/data/nvsr/nvsr68/nvsr68_09_tables-508.pdf

223   https://www.cdc.gov/mmwr/volumes/69/wr/mm6915e3.htm?s_cid=mm6915e3_w

224   https://covid19tracker.health.ny.gov/views/NYS-COVID19-Tracker/NYSDOHCOVID-19Tracker-Fatalities?%3Aembed=yes&%3Atoolbar=no&%3Atabs=n

225   https://www.mdch.state.mi.us/osr/Provisional/MontlyDxCounts.asp#

226   https://www.medrxiv.org/content/10.1101/2020.05.13.20101253v2

227   https://www.worldometers.info/coronavirus/country/us/

228   https://www.thelancet.com/journals/lanpub/article/PIIS2468-2667(20)30089-X/fulltext

229   https://www.foxnews.com/science/third-blood-samples-massachusetts-study-coronavirus

230   https://www.wsmv.com/news/tennessee/almost-750-state-prisoners-test-positive-for-covid-19/article_7466701a-88c1-11ea-99f2-1ffd4312d930.html

231   https://www.reuters.com/article/us-health-coronavirus-prisons-testing-in/in-four-u-s-state-prisons-nearly-3300-inmates-test-positive-for-coronavirus-96-without-symptoms-idUSKCN2270RX

232   https://doc.louisiana.gov/doc-covid-19-testing/

233   https://www.sciencemag.org/news/2020/04/antibody-surveys-suggesting-vast-undercount-coronavirus-infections-may-be-unreliable#

234   https://news.usc.edu/168987/antibody-testing-results-covid-19-infections-los-angeles-county/

235   https://www.washingtonexaminer.com/news/stunningly-high-reported-new-york-infection-rate-illustrates-coronavirus-uncertainty

236   https://www.miamiherald.com/news/coronavirus/article242260406.html

237   https://whyy.org/articles/researchers-at-mits-biobot-use-fecal-matter-to-track-coronavirus-in-delaware/

238   https://www.stripes.com/news/navy/uss-roosevelt-has-nearly-1-000-virus-cases-after-navy-reassesses-how-it-determines-who-s-still-sick-1.627690

239   https://www.stripes.com/news/pacific/asymptomatic-reagan-strike-group-sailors-test-positive-for-coronavirus-after-sequestration-1.627632

240   https://www.wsoctv.com/news/trending/coronavirus-cdc-reviewing-stunning-

universal-testing-results-boston-homeless-shelter/
ZADQ45HCAZEVJAZA3OTCUR7M6M/

241 https://www.nbcnews.com/news/us-news/nearly-900-workers-tyson-foods-plant-indiana-test-positive-coronavirus-n1197776

242 https://www.medrxiv.org/content/10.1101/2020.04.26.20079244v1

243 https://www.n-tv.de/panorama/172-Kontaktpersonen-von-Corona-verschont-article21727469.html

244 https://adc.bmj.com/content/early/2020/05/05/archdischild-2020-319474

245 https://www.nytimes.com/2020/04/15/us/coronavirus-cases-update-live.html

246 https://www.medrxiv.org/content/10.1101/2020.04.26.20079822v1.full.pdf

247 https://www.thelancet.com/journals/lanres/article/PIIS2213-2600(17)30229-1/fulltext

248 https://www.thelancet.com/journals/lancet/article/PIIS0140-6736(20)31142-9/fulltext

249 https://www.cnn.com/2020/04/14/health/social-distancing-research-coronavirus-2022-trnd/index.html

250 https://www.pewresearch.org/fact-tank/2019/09/11/key-findings-about-the-online-news-landscape-in-america/

251 https://www.realclearpolitics.com/articles/2020/05/06/prolonging_the_shutdown_defies_science_and_the_us_constitution_143127.html

252 https://www.realclearpolitics.com/epolls/other/president_trump_job_approval-6179.html

253 https://www.npr.org/sections/health-shots/2020/01/29/800813299/worried-about-catching-the-new-coronavirus-in-the-u-s-flu-is-a-bigger-threat

254 https://www.usatoday.com/story/news/health/2020/01/24/coronavirus-versus-flu-influenza-deadlier-than-wuhan-china-disease/4564133002/

255 https://thehill.com/changing-america/well-being/longevity/480089-coronavirus-sparks-panic-as-flu-poses-greater-threat-to

256 https://www.washingtonpost.com/health/time-for-a-reality-check-america-the-flu-is-a-much-bigger-threat-than-coronavirus-for-now/2020/01/31/46a15166-4444-11ea-b5fc-eefa848cde99_story.html

257 https://www.statnews.com/2020/01/31/as-far-right-calls-for-china-travel-ban-health-experts-warn-coronavirus-response-would-suffer/

258 https://thehill.com/homenews/campaign/481028-biden-slams-trump-for-cutting-health-programs-before-coronavirus-outbreak

259 https://www.azcentral.com/story/news/politics/elections/2020/05/05/joe-biden-rips-president-donald-trump-ahead-his-phoenix-visit/3082396001/

260 https://www.reuters.com/article/us-china-health-who/who-chief-says-widespread-

travel-bans-not-needed-to-beat-china-virus-idUSKBN1ZX1H3

261 https://www.npr.org/sections/health-shots/2020/03/12/815146007/public-health-experts-question-trumps-ban-on-most-travelers-from-europe

262 https://apnews.com/4552fd280d06cf83c63e4cc9b08fe5ce

263 https://thehill.com/policy/transportation/487359-trumps-travel-ban-draws-european-ire-as-crisis-grows

264 https://www.nytimes.com/2020/03/12/world/europe/europe-coronavirus-travel-ban.html

265 https://nypost.com/2020/03/21/blood-on-their-hands-teachers-say-de-blasio-and-carranza-helped-spread-coronavirus/

266 https://www.dailywire.com/news/teachers-blame-de-blasio-schools-chancellor-for-spread-of-coronavirus-the-blood-is-on-their-hands

267 https://www.foxnews.com/media/nbc-news-chuck-todd-trump-blood-on-his-hands

268 https://www.courier-journal.com/story/news/politics/2020/03/17/coronavirus-bill-mcconnell-has-blood-his-hands-candidate-says/5069134002/

269 https://www.inquisitr.com/5974000/donald-trump-blood-hands-president-unfit/

270 https://www.nbcnews.com/politics/donald-trump/pelosi-bashes-trump-coronavirus-president-fiddles-people-are-dying-n1171561

271 https://www.documentcloud.org/documents/6842659-200203-NBCWSJ-April-Poll-4-19-20-Release.html

272 https://www.people-press.org/2020/04/16/most-americans-say-trump-was-too-slow-in-initial-response-to-coronavirus-threat/?utm_source=AdaptiveMailer&utm_medium=email&utm_campaign=20-04-16%20COVID%20Trump_GEN%20DISTRO&org=982&lvl=100&ite=5984&lea=1335245&ctr=0&par=1&trk=

273 https://ourworldindata.org/coronavirus-data?country=USA+HUN+ITA+JPN+ESP+SWE+GBR+FRA+DEU

274 https://hub.jhu.edu/2020/04/07/crystal-watson-roadmap-to-reopen-united-states/

275 https://www.nytimes.com/2003/02/19/opinion/tell-the-truth.html?ref=thomaslfriedman

276 https://www.nytimes.com/2020/04/18/opinion/trump-coronavirus-testing.html?searchResultPosition=5

277 https://www.washingtonpost.com/opinions/2020/04/21/georgia-leads-race-become-americas-no-1-death-destination/

278 https://abcnews.go.com/US/texas-cases-covid-19-increasing-thousands-reopening/story?id=70720497

279 https://www.cdc.gov/mmwr/volumes/69/wr/mm6918e3.htm

280 https://www.mdch.state.mi.us/osr/Provisional/MontlyDxCounts.asp#

281   Authors: Chris Jackson, Mallory Newall, Jinhee Yi; https://www.ipsos.com/en-us/news-polls/abc-news-coronavirus-poll?mod=article_inline

282   https://apnews.com/4e2a20bd01bd2352009c3281b657375d

283   https://www.prnewswire.com/news-releases/64-percent-of-americans-say-theyre-happy-in-their-relationships-300595502.html

284   https://www.psychologytoday.com/us/blog/contemplating-divorce/201709/are-you-among-the-growing-number-unhappy-married-people

285   https://www.ons.gov.uk/peoplepopulationandcommunity/wellbeing/articles/personalandeconomicwellbeingintheuk/whatmattersmosttoourlifesatisfaction#most-important-factors-affecting-life-satisfaction?mod=article_inline

286   https://www.economist.com/graphic-detail/2020/04/22/domestic-violence-has-increased-during-coronavirus-lockdowns

287   https://www.unfpa.org/resources/impact-covid-19-pandemic-family-planning-and-ending-gender-based-violence-female-genital

288   https://www.nbcnews.com/news/us-news/police-see-rise-domestic-violence-calls-amid-coronavirus-lockdown-n1176151

289   https://www.cbsnews.com/news/domestic-violence-additional-31-million-cases-worldwide/

290   https://www.bridgemi.com/children-families/stay-home-dont-stay-safe-domestic-violence-calls-amid-michigan-lockdown

291   https://phys.org/news/2020-06-lockdown-crimes-home-authorities.html

292   https://www.npr.org/sections/coronavirus-live-updates/2020/04/28/847251985/child-sexual-abuse-reports-are-on-the-rise-amid-lockdown-orders

293   http://conference.iza.org/conference_files/Gender_2017/de_cao_e6099.pdf

294   https://time.com/5818006/coronavirus-children-angelina-jolie/

295   https://www.bbc.com/news/world-us-canada-52416330

296   https://www.sbsun.com/2020/04/27/non-violent-crime-drops-in-san-bernardino-during-coronavirus-lockdown/

297   https://www.newstribune.com/news/national/story/2020/apr/12/crime-drops-around-the-world-as-covid-19-keeps-people-inside/824036/

298   https://www.lawenforcementtoday.com/murder-rate-more-than-doubles-in-cincinnati-during-virus-lockdown/

299   https://mynbc15.com/news/nation-world/crime-drops-around-the-world-as-covid-19-keeps-people-inside-04-11-2020-152408165

300   https://www.livemint.com/news/india/covid-19-stay-at-home-reduces-crime-rate-but-fear-of-domestic-violence-rises-11586746861558.html

301   https://www.policeone.com/coronavirus-covid-19/articles/nypd-murders-surge-for-second-week-in-a-row-as-lockdown-continues-YuiA6UaECinHBvSf/

ENDNOTES

302 https://nypost.com/2020/05/18/nyc-shootings-skyrocket-with-dozens-of-victims-in-a-week/

303 https://www.reuters.com/investigates/special-report/health-coronavirus-usa-cost/

304 https://www.wilx.com/content/news/Study-predicts-increase-in-suicide-rates-among-COVID-19-frontline-workers-570016071.html

305 https://www.thelancet.com/journals/lancet/article/PIIS0140-6736(20)30460-8/fulltext

306 https://fox17.com/news/local/feeling-the-pressures-of-the-pandemic-suicide-hotlines-see-800-percent-spike-in-calls

307 https://www.dailymail.co.uk/news/article-8293233/Far-people-Australia-predicted-die-suicide-coronavirus-lockdown.html

308 https://fox17.com/news/local/feeling-the-pressures-of-the-pandemic-suicide-hotlines-see-800-percent-spike-in-calls

309 https://www.graham-center.org/content/dam/rgc/documents/publications-reports/reports/Projected-Deaths-Despair-COVID-19.pdf

310 https://www.census.gov/library/visualizations/2019/comm/largest-school-districts.html

311 https://nypost.com/2020/04/30/study-explores-how-american-parents-are-enduring-covid-19-lockdown-with-their-children/

312 https://networkforpubliceducation.org/wp-content/uploads/2020/04/Teacher-Survey-on-Emergency-Remote-Learning.pdf

313 https://www.theguardian.com/australia-news/2020/may/05/australias-back-to-school-plans-expose-schism-around-children-and-coronavirus

314 https://www.nytimes.com/2020/05/05/health/coronavirus-children-transmission-school.html

315 https://www.sickkids.ca/PDFs/About-SickKids/81407-COVID19-Recommendations-for-School-Reopening-SickKids.pdf

316 https://www.elle.com/culture/career-politics/news/a42336/madonnas-womens-march-speech-transcript/

317 https://news.gallup.com/poll/241634/one-three-americans-felt-urge-protest.aspx

318 https://www.lansingstatejournal.com/story/news/local/2020/04/20/whitmer-responds-critics-says-war-against-conornavirus-requires-sacrifices/5168357002/

319 https://www.michigan.gov/whitmer/0,9309,7-387-90499_90640-527721--,00.html

320 https://www.bridgemi.com/michigan-government/gop-led-legislature-sues-michigan-gov-whitmer-over-emergency-powers

321 https://www.bridgemi.com/michigan-government/gop-led-legislature-sues-michigan-gov-whitmer-over-emergency-powers

322 http://media.graytvinc.com/documents/Restore+Illinois.pdf

323 https://www.scribd.com/document/460677980/Tesla-v-Alameda-County-Complaint-Copy?campaign=SkimbitLtd&ad_group=74968X1582515X09e4cf93e5 f2626c4c20a01a82c94d55&keyword=660149026&source=hp_ affiliate&medium=affiliate

324 https://www.nytimes.com/2020/04/18/us/texas-protests-stay-at-home.html

325 https://www.thelancet.com/journals/lanres/article/PIIS2213-2600(17)30229-1/fulltext

326 https://academic.oup.com/cid/article/65/11/1934/4068747

327 https://www.rcreader.com/commentary/masks-dont-work-covid-a-review-of-science-relevant-to-covide-19-social-policy

328 https://web.archive.org/web/20170512002228/https:/www.oralhealthgroup.com/features/face-masks-dont-work-revealing-review/

329 https://www.nytimes.com/2020/02/29/health/coronavirus-n95-face-masks.html

330 https://www.washingtonpost.com/nation/2020/06/01/americans-are-delaying-medical-care-its-devastating-health-care-providers/?arc404=true

Made in the USA
Middletown, DE
08 August 2020